Silent Journey

L. D. Ross

Best Wishes
Michelle

First Edition – January 2013

ISBN
978-1-4602-1151-9 (Hardcover)
978-1-4602-1152-6 (Paperback)
978-1-4602-1153-3 (eBook)

The author can be reached via e-mail at:
ldrosswriter@telus.net

Produced by:

FriesenPress
Suite 300 – 852 Fort Street
Victoria, BC, Canada V8W 1H8

www.friesenpress.com

Distributed to the trade by The Ingram Book Company

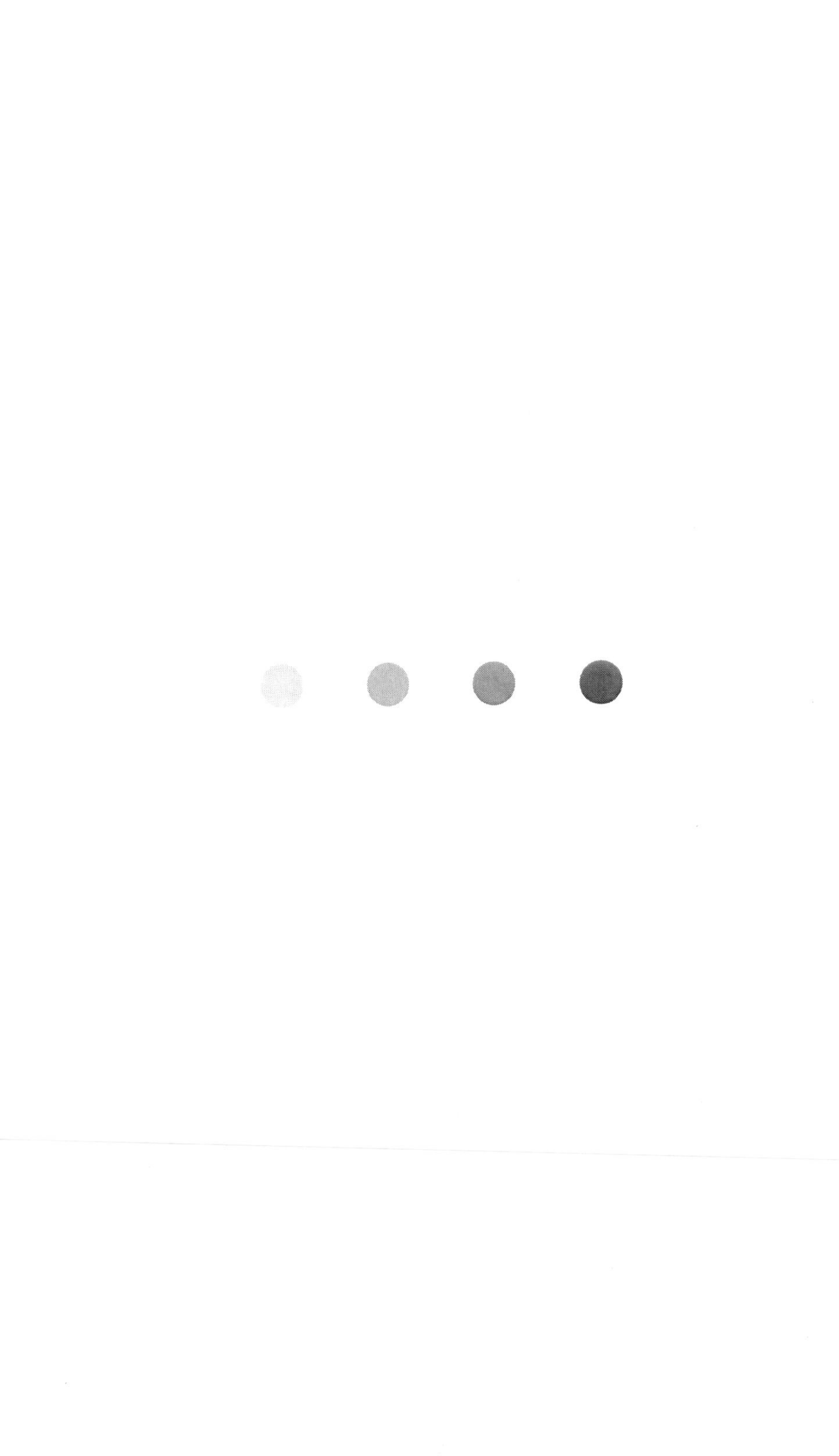

Chapter 1

Michelle and her sister Cori rode together in the white Ford Ranger pickup truck. It was Cori's vehicle; she was driving herself to work at the University of Victoria bookstore. She parked her truck in a parking stall and hopped out.

"See you later," Cori said to her sister. "Good luck at the doctor." She handed Michelle the keys.

"Yeah, no problem," Michelle replied. "See you later." Michelle did not realize that these were the last words she would say to her sister for a very long time.

Michelle entered a nearby building to pay a parking ticket. She had received the ticket a few days earlier. It was a fine for not taking a pay stub from the ticket machine in the first place. At present, she was borrowing Cori's truck so she could visit the campus medical clinic about her persistent headaches.

When Michelle walked back to the truck and hopped into the driver's side, strange things began happening. It was so odd. Her hand was tingling. Had it fallen asleep? She shook it. She flexed her fingers. What an unusual sensation.

The pain in her head had begun five days ago. It was something totally out of the norm. She'd suffered from headaches in the past, but they had always responded to over-the-counter pain relievers.

She tried to lift her arm to place the key in the ignition. This was very weird. Her arm was like rubber, loose and uncontrollable. What was going on? But these headaches were different; the pain was more around the eyes and made worse by light. Bright light was especially uncomfortable. And the agonizing headaches would not stop, no matter what Michelle did. Even at night she slept very little, enduring the constant pain all night long.

Suddenly, an overwhelming weakness invaded her entire body. She panicked. Nothing was working right. It was a terrifying loss of control. Her head felt woozy, fuzzy. Everything was blurring in front of her eyes.

Michelle didn't go to the doctor that often. She'd had a broken arm when she was younger that was placed in a cast, but that was no big deal. The arm was just like new in a matter of a couple of months.

The trees and sky and buildings were swaying in front of her eyes. Thank God she was sitting, for surely she would have fallen right over. Oh, it was awful. *Get help!* she thought to herself. *Honk the horn!*

In her late teens, there had been the problem with stomach cramps. The medical people had tested her with a colonoscopy, but the answer to her problem had finally been discovered by a naturopath. She'd had a simple allergy to pork.

Michelle could no longer comprehend what was going on around her. She was totally confused; overwhelmed. Yes, the horn sounded. Good. Her head was spinning. *Honk the horn.*

Other than that brief episode with the pork allergy, she had always been very healthy and had no need to seek professional medical help. But she needed it now. After a few days with the non-stop headaches, she had finally called her parents to ask for their advice. They encouraged her to see a doctor. And Cori, on that morning, had insisted on it.

It was fortunate for Michelle that there was a security office in the same building where she had just payed her parking ticket. A security employee, a young woman, had heard the alarming horn and ran up to the truck, offering assistance. Michelle never did have a recollection of telling this woman that her sister worked at the bookstore. However, Cori was soon there. Oh, my God, what a relief! Cori was there.

The bookstore was a large building that towered three stories over the adjacent parking lot. In front of the spot where Cori had parked the truck was a grass median separating the parking stalls from the bus terminal. Planted upon this mounded, nicely manicured median were three very young, green leafed maple trees.

Michelle felt her entire body turning on her. The weakness was profound. She was exhausted and frightened. Did someone help her out of the truck? She felt herself in a limp and heavy body. She looked at the thin trunk of a tree. She was crouched on the grass down at the tree's base. A male voice was asking her questions. Did she tell them about her headaches? Did Cori? She closed her eyes. She no longer cared. She no longer had the strength to care. Nausea gripped her insides. Her stomach tightened, and forced its contents onto the young tree.

Then again. And again.

Poor tree, Michelle thought. *Poor little tree.*

• • •

It was reported in hospital records that the "patient" had been found in the University of Victoria parking lot…911 was called for "seizure." First responders found the patient to be alert.

Chapter 2

Michelle was born in the beautiful city of Kamloops, British Columbia on May 28, 1974. She was a lucky little girl to be born in Canada. It is a peaceful country. The quality of life is relatively high compared to a good portion of the world. Most Canadian residents have a decent place to live. Many reside in very comfortable homes, with electric or gas cooking stoves, double door refrigerators, and a gas or oil furnace system to keep them warm and cozy through the long, cold Canadian winters.

Michelle was even more fortunate than a great number of Canadians. She grew up in a supremely desirable location of Canada, the province of British Columbia. Those who live in the prairie provinces flock to the western coastal province of Michelle's birth to spend their summer holidays. British Columbia, or BC, for short, is fondly referred to as every Canadian's playground.

Kamloops is nestled between the Coastal Mountain Range and the majestic Rocky Mountains. It is situated half way between two of Canada's larger and more prosperous cities, Calgary and Vancouver. When travelling by car from either of these two cities Kamloops can only be reached by driving through the high mountain passes, an unnerving experience during a winter storm. However, in the summer, the drive through the mountain passes and the Thompson/Okanagan valley is a breathtaking adventure. One gazes in awe at the sheer enormous size of the rocky peaks and never ever tires of their stunning beauty. Glistening white snow adorns the highest points, sometimes all year around, while tall evergreen trees softly drape the widening bases.

Heading by car down into the valley is thrilling. As one carefully steers along the winding road, ones ears soon plug up from the lowering altitude. The mountains grow shorter in stature, their peaks are more rounded and completely tree covered. Then they slowly evolve into brownish yellow rolling hills that form a base for the life-blood of the valley, the Thompson River. The valley, where Michelle was born, has a moderate climate. It is considered a desert, hot in the summer and cold in the winter. The temperature during the winter hovers around zero Celsius, occasionally dropping ten or twenty degrees below freezing; but not for very long. This lovely area of Canada, where hoards of retirees migrate to escape the brutality of winter, is Michelle's home town. She was, indeed, a fortunate baby.

The first few weeks of Michelle's life were a bit worrisome for her parents. She was born by Caesarean section as were her older sister and, later on, her younger brother. The surgical delivery was booked for a date of two weeks prior to the nine month gestation period. Although she was born a healthy girl, her lungs were not quite fully developed. And this was why little baby Michelle spent the first five days of her life in an incubator.

Young Cori Britton was eighteen months old when she welcomed home her new baby sister. Their mother was unable to breast feed Michelle, which made bottle feeding a part of the daily routine. Because Cori was allowed to feed her sister with the nourishing bottle, a unique bond was established between the two girls, one that granted them the enjoyment of each other as best lifelong friends.

An example of their closeness was when they sometimes dressed the same, as if they were twins. In fact, they thought of themselves as twins, almost inseparable, happily playing together most of the time. They shared the same bedroom "forever." When they got a little older, in high school, they actually looked like twins, and toyed with the idea of switching classrooms. They were quite certain they could fool the teachers; however, they were pretty good girls and thought better of attempting to do this.

All three of the Britton children were good kids. Their parents were proud of their children's scholastic achievements, each of them turning out to be leaders and becoming the valedictorian of their graduating classes. The children seemed to somehow excel to the top, even though their father thought they could be shy at times. They all came through secondary school, Westsyde School, where there were approximately 120 students per grade. Michelle's father, the vice principal of Kamloops High (a much larger school), thought that a smaller number of students definitely meant an advantage for his children; it was easier for them to shine amongst the smaller number of competing students.

Music was an important activity within the Britton household. Michelle's father, Gordon Britton, started playing piano when he was five years old and, in later years, acquired his ARCT in the pipe organ. He spent six years with the Anglican Church as an organist. Cori took up to grade six in piano.

Michelle, however, was not the type of person to stick to any one thing for long. She made an attempt with the piano but "wasn't too keen on it," according to her dad. When she was about five years old she gave guitar a try. Being left handed, though, posed a problem. The teacher had to reverse the strings on the guitar and young Michelle made a brief effort before carrying on to another challenge. The family consensus about Michelle was that she wanted to try everything, but would rarely stick with anything for long. In her elementary school age years she had short-lived experiences with piano lessons, guitar lessons, dance, gymnastics, and tap dancing. Coming from a cold climate, she did have a greater involvement in popular winter sports such as snow skiing and ice skating. Michelle's parents felt they had given her the opportunity to experience a wide variety of things, and Michelle took advantage of these mind expanding adventures.

It was Cori who seemed to embrace the long-term study of her hobbies. Cori was the child who endured years of determined practicing, possibly because of the parental expectations of the first born. She achieved high results. Yet, in Cori's thinking, Michelle was the one who inspired her through every step of her life. Cori referred to her sister as an "amazingly talented individual."

To Cori, Michelle was truly a special child.

• • •

The University of Victoria is designed with a circular road that leads to various buildings inside and outside this paved and curbed thoroughfare. The grounds are lush with well-manicured lawns and mature trees. There is a large parking lot between the Campus Bookstore where Cori had once worked and the Security Building where Michelle had walked to pay her parking ticket. On a grassy knoll between the parking lot and the bus terminal, at the time of Michelle's incident, had been a newly planted deciduous tree. Although no one knows for sure, this is most likely the place where Michelle was laid down by the paramedics for her initial emergency care.

Chapter 3

The University of Victoria Bookstore was where Cori Britton had worked a casual job for the last few years of her studies at the university. After Cori completed her education, she had spent about a year in South Korea then returned to Canada to work in several areas. She did some teaching to adult learners at the Pacific International College. She was a substitute teacher at various schools around Victoria, mostly at Oak Bay Secondary. And she began working again at the UVic bookstore.

Michelle had accompanied Cori to work that sunny morning because Michelle needed Cori's truck to drive herself over to the nearby medical clinic. When Cori had finally insisted that her sister consult a doctor about the relentless headaches she had been having, she was relieved that Michelle had finally listened. The girls were living together in a townhouse near the university. They had been separated for nearly four years, Cori living in Victoria and Michelle doing her thing in Kamloops. Cori felt weird being without her sister. Eventually they could no longer deal with their long term separation. Michelle moved out to the island to be with her best friend.

Cori drove into the parking lot and got out to go to work. Michelle was to then drive the truck over to the clinic.

It was about fifteen minutes later when someone rushed into the bookstore and frantically asked Cori if she owned a white truck. All Cori had heard in the beginning of her working day was the familiar sounds of customers moving about the store, the clanging and ringing of the cash register and the front doors groaning as they opened and closed. She did not hear the desperate honking of a horn from the parking lot. When told to come outside, Cori dashed outdoors to find her sister sitting in the driver's seat of the truck, her body limp and slumped forward.

"Michelle, can you hear me?" Cori whispered to her sister.

Cori gently lifted her sister's drooping head and pushed her shoulders back into the seat. Michelle was drooling saliva everywhere. Cori was too busy tending to her sister to notice that her own heart was racing; that her own breathing was laboured and rapid.

"Michelle, are you okay?" Cori was yelling now, terrified with her sister's non-reaction.

Someone told Cori that an ambulance was on the way. Hearing this news was slightly calming. She studied Michelle's eyes. They were blank and unfocussed. They were barely open, and it seemed as if they were not seeing anything. It appeared to Cori that her sister was having some kind of seizure.

Within minutes help arrived. Emergency medical professionals took over the situation. Time seemed to stand still. The moment was a confusing blur to Cori. She doesn't remember Michelle ever being on the ground or vomiting on the little tree. But she does recall feeling like everything was going to be okay. People were taking care of Michelle now.

Soon the sirens screamed and the ambulance raced towards the hospital that was fortunately only ten minutes away. Cori jumped into her truck and, in a stupor, followed, her body going into autopilot, hands gripping the steering wheel, foot working the clutch. She didn't even think about what she was doing. All she could think about was her sister, her almost twin. Michelle. Michelle was in trouble.

Looking back on this moment in time over eleven years ago, neither Cori nor Michelle remembers the full details of what had happened that day. It was one of those bewildering emergency events of major confusion. The happenings of those few minutes were distorted and surreal and would forever be dissolved into a jumbled nightmare.

And so the waiting began. Michelle had been taken to the Royal Jubilee Hospital. At first Cori didn't bother contacting any relatives or friends. She was expecting information from the doctors. But news about Michelle's condition would not soon be forthcoming. A nurse spoke briefly to Cori, letting her know that Michelle was being examined by the doctors; that so far there was uncertainty about what was happening with her. A while later a male doctor discussed with Cori that they were concerned Michelle may have had something serious happen to her, possibly a stroke, and they would be transferring her to Victoria General Hospital (VGH) where she would have the best care possible. Cori was then allowed a brief visit with Michelle. The doctor prepared her for what she was about to see.

When Cori entered the emergency room she did not like that Michelle was exposed visually to everyone around. There was no privacy. She knew Michelle would not be happy with that. Cori stood at the foot of the bed. There were "a million tubes" attached to Michelle. It was upsetting. How could this be happening? She moved to the left side of the bed. Cori liked being with her sister at that moment. It felt comforting to hold her warm, delicate hand; the dainty fingers; the well- manicured, stylish nails. She bent over her sister and placed a long, delicate kiss on her forehead.

"Everything will be alright." she quietly assured her sister.

Cori was not allowed to spend very much time with Michelle. The doctors were anxious to speedily transfer her to VGH. When Cori left the emergency room she resumed the waiting. This would be the main focus in her life for the next four days. She felt a bit hopeless, helpless, and suddenly very lonely. And yet, she had faith that all would be fine. It couldn't be anything that bad, could it?

Cori could no longer do this alone. She needed her mom. She needed her dad. Maybe Grandma Britton could come and stay with her, even though the elderly woman was in her mid-eighties. There was a phone in the waiting area. Cori called her grandmother. Effie Britton said she would meet Cori as soon as she could get there. Cori felt somewhat relieved. Someone, anyone, to lean on at this moment would help calm her frazzled nerves. She then contacted Tammi, Michelle's best friend. Tammi was working but said she would try to get off early and come to the hospital.

It was a very confusing and stressful time. Did Grandma Britton meet her at the first hospital, or later on at the next hospital? She could not remember. Soon, she was told that Michelle was being transported to VGH and she was to go to General Admitting there. While outside the hospital, she used her cell phone to dial her parent's home number in Kamloops. She could get no answer from home, so dialed her mom's work number. She was put on hold and waited quite a while on the phone; then her mother's concerned voice finally answered.

Cori couldn't restrain her emotions. She blurted out the bad news through a torrent of tears. "They think Michelle has had a stroke," she told her mother. "She's going downhill fast. Please come. Please come." Cori had been terribly afraid this awful news would create an uncontrollable panic with her parents. She could imagine them "totally freaking out" and having an accident on the roads driving to Victoria. She was surprised that her mom was very calm and "nurse-like." It was actually quite reassuring.

When Cori arrived at Victoria General she was escorted into a very small room. It was so crowded, in fact, that if two people sat across from one another their knees would almost touch. In this room were a couch, one chair, and a phone. She could tell by the nurse's somber face that something bad had happened. Cori sat in the chair and wrapped her arms around herself. She was cold. She felt numb, disbelieving. She sat in the chair for hours, staring straight forward, waiting for more news, waiting for someone, a friend or a family member, to be with her.

• • •

Cori and Michelle had experienced some great times over the years. The girls shared the same bedroom throughout the majority of their childhood years. They had such fun together, making up little stories and laughing and giggling in their beds until all hours, about the most ridiculous things. They enjoyed countless hours together, actively building stuff with their Lego toys, or quietly lying in their beds, reading their books.

They loved watching movies, one of their favorite being *The Pirate Movie* starring Kris Kristofferson. The sisters were quite the singing team as they taped the songs of this musical spoof and transcribed the words so they could learn them.

The family had a place on Shuswap Lake where the girls practically lived on the water. They were two kids with not a care in the world, bobbing along on their huge air tube, riding the waves caused by passing boats. Often, they would try to knock one another off the tube, screaming and laughing and carrying on for hours and hours.

A family tradition was the entire Britton gang gathering together on Saturday nights to watch Hockey Night in Canada. Cori and Michelle would lie on the floor in front of the wood burning fireplace, just relaxing, enjoying the warmth of the fire, content with the family, content with each other.

• • •

A doctor, clipboard in hand, pulled up a chair in front of Cori and introduced himself. He was the neurologist dealing with Michelle. He asked all sorts of questions. Had Michelle bumped her head recently? Had she fallen at some time? A minor car accident? How long did she complain of headaches? So many questions. It would take serious thought over a period of time before Cori would piece together the series of events that may or may not have caused Michelle's medical problem. She was so young. It just didn't make sense. As long as Cori could remember, Michelle had perfect health. When Michelle was in grade school, a play friend had jumped off the teeter totter and Michelle had broken her arm from the fall. Cori remembered the cast. It was no big deal.

Headaches weren't something Michelle had ever complained about. Cori did recall one time when Michelle was working in Banff and had been bothered with a migraine, but it had only lasted one day, and was soon forgotten. During the month before Michelle's hospitalization, however, Cori had definitely noticed peculiar things happening with her sister. Unlike their normal relationship, where the two sisters rarely fought, and made up quickly from disagreements, Cori and Michelle had been fighting "like cats and dogs." This unusual friction worried Cori, but she had chalked it up to them being in the "wrong headspace" at that moment in time and possibly needing some space apart.

Cori recalls, "I remember I was going through a hard time, thinking about many things in my own life and often grumpy, not wanting to talk to many others…and she was doing her own thing, but we were never far from one another nor ever really upset at each other. So we did talk about a few things and it was best, in this instance, to be 'agreeing to disagree.' That seemed to calm our disputes down and I think that led to her finally going to the doctor."

There were other things Cori remembered. Michelle "stole" her truck on a couple of occasions. The agreement between the girls was that Michelle could borrow Cori's truck any time she wanted as long as she asked first. That was the agreement. And it was unlike Michelle to just take the vehicle without permission. That had never happened before. That was such odd behavior for Michelle. In the past Michelle would always have asked, and Cori would always have said "sure."

When Cori gave it serious thought, she came to realize that Michelle's personality had been different. It had changed a bit.

Now, sitting in the hospital, anxiously waiting for news, any news, on her sister, Cori realized that Michelle's recent peculiar behavior was beginning to have an explanation; now it made some sense.

• • •

In the Emergency Centre of the hospital, doctors wrote: 'Would open eyes to voice and move right side to commands. Zero verbal response. Neck supple. Lungs clear. Vomiting in ER. Weak withdrawal to pain. Patient intubated.'

Michelle was given the medications Pavulon, Versed, and Fentanyl. Pavulon is used to relax the muscles, a means to eliminate spontaneous breathing, allowing the patient to adjust to mechanical ventilation. Versed is typically used for sedation during procedures that do not require general anesthesia, but can also be used to keep a patient calm while on a ventilator. Fentanyl is an opioid often used to treat pain.

Dr. W. E. Martin, the attending neurologist, wrote that Michelle 'was found in her own vehicle at UVic parking lot complaining of dizziness and nausea, and then became unconscious before (responder's) arrival. There was no witnessed seizure activity.'

• • •

Obviously, there were conflicting reports on the condition of Michelle during the onset of her emergency. This confusion may have been caused by the growing number of people involved in her care. And Michelle may have moved in and out of consciousness throughout the ordeal of ambulance transport and hospital emergency procedures.

Sandy Fulton was the social worker who assisted families and patients in the intensive care and neurology sections of Victoria General. She'd had a long career there and had developed a keen sense of understanding the many emotions people go through in an emergency situation. She first saw Michelle in intensive care. "She was in a desperate kind of situation. She needed ICU support. I believe she was intubated, meaning she was on a breathing machine, and there were grave concerns for her survival."

• • •

On May 19 Cori wrote this in her personal diary: *Gosh! Unbelievable. I don't know how else to describe this. Michelle, dear little sister, is in the hospital, in the Intensive Care Unit. She is hooked up to a breathing apparatus (for her protection), has a tube down her nose as well to suck up her stomach contents. She is hooked up to a machine that monitors her heartbeat, etc. and blood pressure. Plus she has intravenous for various drugs. It's unbelievable!! I'm here sitting in the lounge/waiting room. Dr. Wan, Dr. Martin, Dr. Waters, Dr. Campbell, Ann, Shelagh, Kim, Joey, Peter….The list goes on and on. Everybody who has helped; who is helping. I can't believe I'm documenting something like this. It is truly an episode right from ER. Only this episode has the potential to run a whole season. Who knows!?*

Chapter 4

The three children amused themselves on the swings in the Stuart Wood Elementary school yard. There were two boys. One little boy was three years old, the other four years of age. Playing along with the two boys was a four year old girl. Joan Britton, the children's caregiver that day, tried on most days to get the children outside for a while, weather permitting. The playground was about two blocks away from Kamloops Immigrant Services, where Joan was a child care worker. Her job was caring for preschool children while their immigrant parents studied English as a second language. It was a typically warm sunny morning in Kamloops and, as usual in the Thompson Okanagan valley, the skies were clear blue and the summer heat was already felt in the constant breeze. That particular day, however, May 17, 1999, would change Joan's life forever. Joan is Michelle's mother.

Joan's place of birth was Edmonton, Alberta, home of the famous Edmonton Oilers and Wayne Gretsky. Her mother, Edna Mary Holland, and her father, Cyril "Cy" George Emery, were both also born in Edmonton. When Joan was 2 years old her family moved to West Vancouver and that is where Joan grew up. It was a small family. Joan had only one sibling, a younger brother. It was obviously a stable family, as Edna and Cy lived in the same house for 56 years. Cy Emery worked as a motor vehicle parts person and had a good job as Parts Manager for Clarke Simpkins Limited, a car dealership in Vancouver. Joan remembers a good childhood. Edna, who was a stay at home mom, took her children out on most days: shopping or to the beach at Ambleside or to playschool. Edna babysat some of the neighborhood children, so Joan remembers having lots of playmates. Where the Emery family lived was across the street from Leyland Park, a municipal park of a few acres. There was a big rock on this playground that the kids could climb and play on. The rock was also a lookout over the entrance to Vancouver Harbor and Stanley Park. It was beautiful spot. A common game for kids to play in those days was Cowboys and Indians. Joan thought of herself as a bit of a tomboy, always enjoying an active playtime. Because her home was on a hill, she also had a great time sledding down the lane and road in the snow.

In her teen years, Joan had lots of girlfriends and had an active social life after school and on weekends. She did a lot of babysitting after she turned the age of 13. During high school, Joan and some of her friends went to St. Paul's Hospital once a week to be candy stripers. Joan was well educated. She completed her 13 years of primary education and then studied to become Registered Nurse. She was the only one of all the girls to continue on into a nursing career. As a young woman, Joan could not know how critically important her chosen career would be in her future.

• • •

Joan noticed that the secretary of Stuart Wood had come out to the playground and was waving at her. There was a phone call for her; it was her daughter, Cori. That was very odd. Cori had never before called her at work. The secretary explained that Cori had gotten the school's phone number from someone at Joan's workplace. Joan felt a twinge of anxiety, wondering what this could be about. She dashed into the school, the secretary quickly gathering up the children behind her. When Joan answered the phone, it was not difficult to pick up on the panic in Cori's voice. Words at this point took second place to emotion. "Mom. It's Michelle," Cori blurted out through gasping sobs. "She was in the truck. And she was trying to get help. And they got me. And she isn't moving. Her eyes are…"

Joan used her most reassuring voice to try to calm her daughter. She needed information. She asked questions. Cori answered. Being a mother had prepared Joan for emergencies. Children were always getting into one scrape or another. She knew that maintaining an authoritative, controlled demeanor would be best for a shaken Cori. So, Joan stifled her own increasing anxiety and became almost businesslike. Get the facts. Make a plan. Calm the kid. It was fortunate for Joan that there were now so many things to quickly do. She had very little time to sit and ponder the worst of thoughts that often can invade a person's mind. At this stressful, chaotic time, it did not once occur to her that Michelle could die.

Joan hurried the children back to Kamloops Immigrant Services and informed her boss of the situation. She asked for some time off work. She phoned her friend, Helen Gulley, who agreed to fill in for her at work. There was no question that she would be going to Victoria. Within minutes she was in her car and heading home.

During the 15 or 20 minute drive home, Joan's mind was trying to sort out what she could do. There wasn't a flight from Kamloops to Victoria until 3 o'clock in the afternoon. And then, Joan thought, if they caught a flight they wouldn't have a vehicle to drive once down there. She had tried to call Gordon at home, but there was no answer. This didn't cause her concern. She knew that Gordon and her son, Paul, had planned to go out to the lake to do something out there. When she arrived home she checked out the back door to see if Gordon and Paul had not yet left for the lake. Luckily, they were still in the back yard working together on a water feature. She was relieved when she could allow her own anxiety to show. She gave Gordon the little information she knew.

Years later, Joan would reflect on her good fortune that her husband and son had changed their minds on their lake activities that day.

So, decisions had to be made. She and Gordon agreed that driving to Victoria would be the best plan. Because Victoria is located on Vancouver Island, some distance over water, she was well aware of the long drive and equally long ferry ride ahead of them.

Cori had called home to tell her parents that Michelle was being transported by ambulance to VGH, which specialized in neurology. Within half an hour the two nervous parents had eaten a quick lunch, packed two suitcases and a snack, and were on the road to Victoria. Joan and Gordon were accustomed to this scenic drive through the Coastal Mountains. Several times a year they ventured out to Victoria to visit family: Gordon's mother, a cousin and, of course, Cori and Michelle.

The drive from Kamloops to Vancouver took a few hours. Joan and Gordon talked some about what could be happening to their daughter, though, for the most part, they were quiet and thoughtful. They may have even mentioned the possibility of Michelle dying, but they decided it was best to be positive in their thinking. Joan prayed. A lot. Then there was the wait for the Tsawassen Bay ferry that carries countless numbers of cars and trucks across the Strait of Georgia to Vancouver Island. Several ferries cross this stretch of water every day, the last one leaving in the early evening. Joan and Gordon arrived at the ferry terminal just in time to load onto the last ferry of the day.

Normally this would be a picturesque, peaceful journey. That day, though, darkness had already shadowed the pristine waters, and a solemn mood hovered over the worried couple. They talked a little bit more about what may have happened to Michelle. They discussed their mutual concern. But mostly, they were simply shocked and confused about this unexpected turn of events in their lives. For a large part of their journey they sat on the gently swaying ship, staring in stunned silence out the ship's windows into the blackness, wondering what could possibly have happened to their young daughter. Joan prayed that Michelle would at least live until she had gotten a chance to see he; tell her she loved her. Sometime during Joan's prayers a sense of calm came over her: everything would be alright. Michelle would live.

Joan and Gordon finally arrived at the Intensive Care Unit of the VGH at 9:30 p.m. They met Cori in the waiting area. The strain on her face revealed intense worry along with relief that her mom and dad were now there. Joan could tell that her oldest daughter was completely drained. She held Cori tightly for a moment, reassuring her that she was no longer alone in her struggle.

The family immediately went into the ICU. Joan was not at all disturbed by the surroundings. Her nursing experience over the years had given her a familiarity with the various machines attached to her daughter by an assortment of plastic tubes. Lying in Bed A in the ICU, Michelle had an airway tube in her mouth that was giving her oxygen through a ventilator. There was a gastric tube in Michelle's nose that went down into her stomach. There was an intravenous needle placed into her arm. A heart monitor was connected to her chest. A finger clamp was attached to her finger, constantly monitoring Michelle's pulse. A blood pressure cuff was wrapped around Michelle's arm, taking her blood pressure every 10 or 15 minutes. To Joan, Michelle seemed semi-conscious. Her eyes were closed. Joan was told that Michelle had received a small amount of morphine and a muscle relaxant, and also medications to settle her stomach.

Joan moved up to her daughter's bedside and touched her hand. She whispered in Michelle's ear, "Mom and dad are here." Joan absolutely knew that her daughter could hear her voice. The unconscious girl seemed to immediately relax in the presence of her parents. However awful it was for a mother to see her child in such mortal danger, Joan, for a brief moment, felt peaceful inside.

In a short while the family left Michelle's room. Joan collapsed in a chair and wept. She realized that Cori had definitely not overreacted to her sister's condition. This was very, very serious. Privately, Joan said many thank you prayers, thankful that Michelle was in good hands in a good hospital, thankful that Michelle was still alive.

From what she had seen in the ICU, Joan was mindful that Michelle was gravely ill. The thought of losing her feisty girl was too awful to imagine. It seemed like not so long ago that her blue eyed, white-blond little daughter was challenging the wisdom of her parents. Many years ago, the family had been visiting Michelle's aunt's place in Ohio, swimming in the pool. Determined young Michelle insisted on removing her water wings. She was making such a scene. Joan and Gordon eventually gave in. They removed the air-filled water balloons from Michelle's tiny arms. They allowed the stubborn little girl to attempt swimming on her own. And down she went. Onlookers were aghast, but the Brittons knew what they were doing. It was a lesson Michelle needed to learn. Michelle realized the hard way that she couldn't keep her head above water on her own. Her dad promptly came to her rescue. And she no longer argued with mom and dad. She definitely had learned her lesson.

Michelle was a fun child. When she was really young she was a typical toddler. Her first word was "mom." She had a common childhood habit of twirling her hair. She played with stuffed teddy bears and rode a tricycle, then a bicycle. She displayed all the expected behaviors of a little girl. Joan thought fondly of when she, Michelle, Cori, and their friend Diane were all lined up in the kitchen cutting the ends off beans. The girls had had so much fun that day. Oh, and camping and boating and dressing up for Halloween, all such fun. Joan had always maintained her role as parent, yet still enjoyed the antics of the children.

But when Michelle grew older and more independent, her parents were often caught off guard by Michelle's spontaneous adventures. Joan was occasionally concerned about her youngest daughter. Alcohol, cigarette smoking and drugs seemed not a worrying issue, however, Michelle became involved at a young age, sixteen, with a teenager named Wes who she was tutoring in math. He was little younger than her. Wes was heavily into hockey and was determined to follow his dream of one day playing for the NHL. The two teens developed a very close relationship. Joan and Gordon, at that time, didn't think Michelle and Wes "as an item" was the best thing. Joan thought Wes was a very nice young fellow, and he had good parents. The problem was, of course, their very young ages, and also Wes's focus on the hockey which, to Joan and Gordon, would take the him nowhere in the future. And, in the minds of Joan and Gordon, a good future for Michelle was imperative.

When Michelle was in her late teens, Joan knew that her daughter was more into drinking alcohol that her two siblings. Even though Michelle was not entirely forthcoming to her parents with information on her questionable social activities, Joan knew much more than young Michelle realized. When Michelle entered adulthood, however, she became more and more independent. Joan came to expect surprises, as in the time when Michelle called her up one day, asked if her mom was sitting down, and subsequently announced that she and a few friends were, at the spur of the moment, flying off to Hawaii. Also, in regards to flying, Joan and Gordon knew very well that Michelle was keenly interested in flying an airplane herself. They had consistently encouraged her to put off flying lessons until she had completed her university education. Unbeknownst to Joan and Gordon, Michelle had already flown a few times.

That was Joan's unstoppable Michelle.

• • •

When Michelle was examined by neurologist, Dr. Martin, he noted 'she is well nourished, no signs of trauma. Neck is not stiff.

Eardrums are normal. Thyroid normal. Chest, heart, and abdomen are all normal. She is seemingly unconscious but I note that she did respond when we did a lumbar puncture. There is no active movement of her extremities.'

The fluid from Michelle's lumbar puncture was clinically clear. There was a CT scan of her head, and an electroencephalogram (ECG) done. A drug screen was obtained.

Dr. Martin pondered the causes of his young patient's condition. He thought encephalitis was a possibility. A flagrant meningitis or subarachnoid hemorrhage had already been excluded through tests. He also wondered if she had had a seizure and was Postictal (the term for a patient's state after they've had a seizure). But he thought this was unlikely as she had been in this condition for much longer than usual for a Postictal patient. The possibility of a drug effect was being considered and appropriate testing was underway. Dr. Martin noted: 'This is a somewhat mysterious problem.'

• • •

Sandy Fulton, the hospital social worker, took charge of Michelle's family. "I usually try to start at a really practical place because the family doesn't know me," she later explained. Sandy would see if she could develop a rapport with the family and would begin with practical issues. Where was the family staying? She would discuss with them issues of parking, transportation and places to eat. Even insurance was mentioned. When the family felt more comfortable, Sandy would then help them with the more emotional side of the emergency. This part of the process would be different with the various types of people Sandy dealt with. Some remained more private in their thoughts, while others would quickly embrace her help with their feelings. Sandy would start talking to them, asking how they were doing. She would ask what kinds of information they needed. She wanted to know if they were having good communications with physicians and nursing staff. What did they need from all of their caregivers? Would they like to have a family conference so they could meet with the physician and nursing staff that were currently helping their child? Sandy would further say to the family, "Do you have any questions? If you have any questions, write them down. If it's two o'clock in the morning and you can't sleep and you have a burning question, write it down because you're probably not going to remember what that question was in the morning." Those kinds of things.

It was Sandy who suggested to Joan and Gordon that they keep a daily diary. "It gives family something to do because most of the time at that situation they just don't know what to do and they're at a loss for how they can help," she explained.

Chapter 5

Gordon Britton and his son Paul were in the back yard, beginning work on a water feature. They were discussing how, from the top of a rock wall, they would create a waterfall that would wind its way down to a fish pond at the flat level of the lawn. A pump would keep the water gently flowing over the rocks, creating the peaceful sound that only mother-nature's music can do. Father and son were happy as clams gathering the needed materials, totally enjoying their shared project. Initially, they had planned to go out to the lake, but the work out there wasn't pressing and they had decided they were "not keen on a long drive" that day. They certainly did not expect the back door of the house to open and see a very distressed Joan anxiously calling out to them.

It was fortunate for Gordon and Joan that both of them responded well in emergencies. They worked like a well-rehearsed team. Once Joan had told her husband of Michelle's situation, they made a plan together, organized the trip to Victoria, and, with adrenaline-pumped energy, were ready to get going.

Gordon was not the type of man to get rattled when faced with a frightening problem. He accepted the fact that whatever had happened to Michelle was serious. He knew he and Joan had to get to Victoria as soon as they could, but he also realized that there was only so much speed possible. No matter how fast they wanted to get there, it always took a certain amount of time to travel to Victoria, and there was no getting around that.

Gordon was the driver. And it was a good thing that he assumed this responsibility, for he knew he would be impatient and critical as a passenger. Concentrating on the road distracted his mind from the reason he was on the move. He and Joan discussed the range of medical problems that could have afflicted their youngest daughter. They also talked about their responsibilities at home. Although Gordon was retired, Joan still had a job where parents relied on and trusted her to care for their pre-school aged children. And then there were the household things: security, bills, appointments, meetings. So much to think of. The thought of Michelle dying did momentarily creep into Gordon's mind. He imagined it could be a brain issue - encephalitis, an aneurism, a stroke. At this point he could do nothing but hope she would be okay.

• • •

When Gordon was a child, his family was closely involved with the Oak Bay United Church, a wonderful place that was the center of much of their lives. Horace and Effie, Gordon's parents, were in the church choir, and taught Sunday school. Horace also managed the construction of an adjacent hall to the church building. Best of all was their membership in the Couples Club where they developed lifelong friends. Oak Bay is a smaller municipality, one of 12 municipalities making up Greater Victoria, on the southern coast of Vancouver Island. It would be fair to say it is one of the most beautiful places in Canada.

Gordon spent most of his childhood, from age 5 to 16, in Oak Bay and in the same house. He and his two neighborhood buds, Terry and Larry, had a great time playing around the neighborhood, spending time together at each other's houses, and riding their bikes all over Oak Bay. Gordon and the two other boys remain friends to this day.

Horace Britton built a 10 foot plywood boat when Gordon was about 12 years old. Gordon remembers many happy experiences in and around the waters of Victoria and the Gulf Islands. From that first boat, Gordon was hooked and made certain there was always a boat in his life, with lots and lots of fun on the water.

Music was a constant part of Gordon's life. He began classical piano lessons as a young boy and continued his musical studies throughout his school years. At the age of 14 Gordon travelled by bike after school every day to St. John's Anglican Church downtown to practice organ lessons on the large five-manual pipe organ. Throughout Gordon's life he has been involved in some way with the church. He played organ for the Anglican Church for six years.

Gordon was well-educated, acquiring his Bachelor of Arts, a teaching diploma, and his Masters of Arts. At this point in Gordon's life, now that he had completed his education, he felt he needed a change. Even though Victoria had given him a lifetime of great memories, it was time to move on to new experiences; to venture from his home on the island to the more industrious mainland. His first choice would have been to move to the Southern Interior of BC, preferably Kelowna. However, back in 1963, there was little growth or opportunity in that area. Gordon had a friend from university who wanted to go to the North Thompson where there may have been some teaching jobs. He and his friend went to a job fair at UBC, a "cattle market" as they referred to it in those days. Gordon was not overly thrilled with Kamloops on his first visit. His brand new Chrysler Valiant convertible was covered in silt in a matter of minutes. He had a conversation with the Superintendent of Schools, a fellow musician, who was looking for a music teacher. And, despite Gordon's disgust with the dry, windy city of Kamloops, he accepted a teaching job there that was to be his career until he retired.

Now that he was settled and his career was in place, the only thing Gordon was missing was a girlfriend. He and a few other teachers were complaining that they weren't meeting any eligible, single young women. One of the teachers was married to a nurse and, eventually, they arranged a meeting for him with three of her single nurse colleagues. They all met for a drink at a local bar. Of course, Joan was the best looking and most attractive of the three ladies. She seemed to Gordon a discreet, sensitive, and sensible young lady. She was not brash, loud, or boisterous. She was quiet and courteous. Gordon loved that about her.

Meeting Joan was the beginning of a happy successful family life. Joan was also involved with the church, having an Anglican background. Gordon had a history with the United Church. When Gordon and Joan were married about a year later they did not do much about the problem of the type of church they would attend. It was not until they were invited by close friends to attend the Kamloops United Church that the young married couple decided this particular church would be a part of their spiritual journey together. At this time their daughters were ages two and four, and baby Paul had not yet been born.

The children's introduction to church was through their parents at the Kamloops United Church Sunday School. Joan led a group of young girls called the Explorers. Along with the church activities, the children would spend a lot of their time with the school choir and the school band. Westsyde School had excellent music and drama programs in those years. Gordon believed that his children's school experience was a good one. His children were well-liked by their fellow classmates and were often looked up to for leadership

In recalling his years as a father, Gordon thought of himself as a friend to his youngsters, yet always maintaining his role as their caregiver and advisor. He thought his children were really good kids. Sure, there were times when the kids would not listen to him, like those times when they were cross-country skiing. Gordon knew if the kids went too far they would be too tired to make their way back. He would tell them they had gone too far and to turn back.

When they paid no mind to his concerns, he would warn them that he would not carry them home. They were typical kids that way.

Gordon thought about what wonderful times the family had when they would go up to Wallaper Lake for a late January winter weekend every year. A few families would get together at a rustic little resort and tough it out with a wood stove, water from an outdoor well, and an outhouse. They all had a marvelous time. When everyone got a little older, they moved on to vacationing at places with a few more comforts such as hot and cold running water. They would often go to the Vernon Lodge and Silver Star Mountain for family winter outings.

Although none of the children, in Gordon's mind, had given their parents any particular grief, Michelle did "present more of a challenge." Michelle was the one who, with her friend Adele, climbed up on the garden shed and dented the roof. It wasn't a major thing to Gordon; just one of those things that kids did. Michelle didn't really get into any serious trouble. However, she was quite spontaneous in her actions. It was Michelle who decided that the family should have a dog. The neighbors around the corner had a litter of mongrel pups they were selling for 15 dollars each. Gordon and Joan were skeptical, but Michelle had decided it was time they had a dog. She brought the pup home and named it Trixie after the popular teen book series, Trixie Belden. Gordon recalled what a joy Trixie was to the family for 12 years until "the little thing died."

The one thing about Michelle that frustrated Gordon was her tendency to quickly tire of the various things she tried. The way he described it was she would "move from this to this to that to this." It was when Michelle grew into her mid- to late teens that Gordon had the odd worry about her. Michelle was beginning to exercise her independence. When Michelle began a relationship with Wes, the young hockey player, Gordon thought it was a bit distracting for both of them to some degree. Gordon knew that Wes had the dream of becoming an NHL star, but Gordon also knew how unlikely that would be. So at times, Gordon and Joan were "a little restless about that relationship." At the age of nineteen, Michelle decided she was going to travel Australia by herself. Gordon was anxious about that, but luckily Michelle was met in Sydney, Australia by associates of her uncle who got her organized for travelling north as far as Cairnes. This was the way it was with Michelle: never a dull moment.

• • •

When Gordon and Joan arrived at the VGH, they made their way to the Intensive Care section of the hospital. They found Cori in the family waiting area. Right away Gordon knew he had to take charge. Cori had been running on adrenaline for 12 hours. She was very upset. Tired. Scared. She had been dealing with this trauma non-stop all day and was clearly needing her parents' support. Gordon realized that Cori was experiencing the fear of losing her best friend in the world. Throughout the years, Michelle and Cori had been "quite inseparable." He held his daughter and comforted her, but mostly he wanted to find out the facts right away. How? What? Why? He was anxious to talk to the doctor in charge. A nurse led Gordon, Joan, and Cori into the ICU.

The ICU is an intimidating place for the average layperson. It is a quiet, serene room. Spotlessly clean. An oval shaped counter at the center of the room serves as a work station for ICU specialists. There are several monitors on the counter, displaying vital signs of the patients. All around the outside edges of the ICU space are eight rooms, each cluttered with all sorts of medical equipment. Each machine is attached to some sort of wire or tube, each with its own vital purpose. There is no privacy in these rooms. The interior walls and entrance doors are all made of glass. Each patient can be seen from all angles at all times. The seriousness of the life and death dramas taking place in this room is disturbingly palpable.

Gordon saw his cute little blue-eyed blond lying in the bed, unconscious. He could tell she was close to death. Now that he was finally there, he could only feel a painful helplessness. He tenderly patted his little girl, held the hands of his family, and tried to comfort them. After a while they left Michelle to rest, returning to the waiting room. This was very frustrating for Gordon. He needed to speak to the neurologist who was in charge of Michelle. He wanted an expert to tell him what had happened to Michelle and to do something to help her. He wanted answers, action.

As they all sat down in the small, enclosed room, Cori passed on what little information she knew: how Michelle had collapsed in the truck after having a sort of seizure, how Michelle was in too critical a condition for the first hospital to deal with her. Gordon criticized the time lost between the two hospitals. He fretted over the time between tests and results. The waiting was unbearable. Finally, around midnight, they all left for the girls' townhouse to attempt some rest and sleep. It would be a long, fitful night.

• • •

The medical investigation continued. Doctors probed all areas of Michelle's and her family's medical history. They asked the family if Michelle had recently been to a chiropractor or masseuse. They questioned the family history of strokes happening at an early age. They wanted to know if there were any problems with high levels of cholesterol with any family members. Did Michelle smoke? Did she drink alcohol?

Everything seemed normal. Michelle did not have a brain tumor. There was no history of a recent trauma. Michelle's complaints of headaches led doctors to consider that she could possibly have had a stroke. Another thought by consulting physician, Dr. Kemble, was that there may have been a dissection of one of Michelle's arteries. He recommended they check with the radiologist for any evidence on the MRI scan of "an occlusion to the basilar or one of the vertebral arteries."

Sandy Fulton, as a social worker, always had a heavy workload. When it came to Michelle, Sandy expressed, "I think I gave her the time that she needed, and not that I would take away from others, but being able to manage time in a situation that…you've got this whole continuum of dead and dying, really needing help…to bus tickets on the other end. So you can prioritize those kinds of things very easily. The most important get the most time."

Sandy could not help but feel for Gordon as she knew it was very difficult for him. "They've got this lovely daughter who's got all kinds of promise. She's going to university. She's soon to graduate. Life is good. And then it got…"

Sandy thought Gordon Britton was a very stoic man, but was caught up in the disbelief that this awful thing could happen. She wondered what he was thinking, if he was already considering the worst. She knew that thoughts could make anybody sick. But she also noticed that Gordon was realistic. Hospital staff would give him information and he would say he understood it, and that maybe he did not agree with it, but he understood. In Sandy's eyes he played the tough guy, at least on the outside.

Chapter 6

Paul was the youngest of the Britton children. He often felt like he lived in the shadow of his two older sisters. He was the "third wheel", probably because of the age differences. The girls were quite close in age, while Paul was much younger; and his physical capabilities were always way behind them. But he worshiped his sisters. As it turned out, Cori and Paul were very like tempered and therefore had a tendency toward sibling bickering. So, "Shell actually became the mediator during these tiffs."

Paul really couldn't remember a lot of childhood events with his sisters or things they shared. If anything, he recounts his experience was more like being "dragged along" when the three of them did things. He didn't feel he had ever been "engaged in my big sister's life." It was only in later years when they all became young adults that Paul became closer to Michelle and Cori.

There were two vacations that Paul remembered well: Hawaii and Disneyland. Paul's grandparents joined the family on both of these trips. Paul enjoyed his holiday but, because of the age difference between him and the girls, he mostly played with his grandparents and his mom and dad. Cori and Michelle did their own thing and were thick as thieves.

There was one time in Hawaii when the girls participated in surfing lessons. Paul really wanted to join them but he was too little. He had to stay back, had to suffer watching his sisters in the surf while he was stuck on the beach making sand castles and digging holes in the sand.

As the children grew a little older the whole family toured across Canada and explored the Maritimes. Paul tried, but couldn't get into the antics of *Anne of Green Gables.* His sisters, however, were addicted to the novels, especially having visited Prince Edward Island where the story originated. All they wanted to do was read. Paul, once again, was not included. They were older. He was younger. They were girls. He was a boy.

It was during a trip to Europe with Michelle and their parents that Paul spent more time with his younger sister. Cori had not come along. Paul and Michelle became travelling buddies. There were a few experiences that he would never forget. He so enjoyed travelling along in their rented Passat Wagon listening to the music of Right Said Fred. And the spas in the Black Forest were especially soothing and majestic.

The weirdest event was Paul's first legitimate beer in Heidelberg with his dad and mom and sister. The most awesome time was their stay at a Swiss farm house outside Lucerne. There was an evening fireworks show that Paul and Michelle watched from their bedroom window. Then there was a parade of boats going back to their moorings on Lake Lucerne after the fireworks ended. As they commonly shared a room during their travels, Paul and Michelle experienced a lot of things together. It was a time when they would get to know each other.

At home, there were many uncomfortable times with Michelle. Paul often found himself a bystander witnessing the fights between Michelle and her parents. Her high school years, in particular, were a difficult time for Michelle. She often had to do things the difficult way. Eventually she grew out of her rebellious stage, but not before "sowing her wild oats."

When Paul enrolled in the University of Victoria, he shared a townhouse with Cori, Michelle and their friend, Tammi. Every summer Paul would go home to Kamloops to "work and play and save money for the next year's adventure at university." Paul and his family had more connections in Kamloops, so it was easier for him to land a job there. He had a girlfriend now, Jenn. They had been dating for about a year and a half.

• • •

The day of Michelle's emergency, Paul was working with his dad on their outdoor waterfall project. This was always a wonderful time for Paul. He and his dad often worked on stuff together. It was a time when father and son would join together and bond their relationship. When Paul first heard of Michelle's problem he didn't know what to think. It was the first family emergency in his life. It was sort of a blur, rushing to put away the tools, observing his parent's frantic packing, and watching them fly out the door. Paul was forced to deal with the frightening situation by himself as his parents had asked him to hold down the fort.

Paul wanted to distract himself from negative thoughts. He called a couple of his close friends and asked them to bring over a movie. He needed the company. He ordered a pizza. Frank, Paul's very good friend, was "awesome and sensitive to the wave of emotions I was experiencing." His other friend seemed oblivious to the news of his sister. Paul found that interesting, how different people reacted to these types of situations.

There was a "ton of stuff" going through Paul's mind. That night, alone in his bed and removed from his immediate family, dealing with a crisis all on his own, Paul cried for his sister.

One time in the past, when Paul was in grade 12, his dad left him in charge of the house while his parents went on a vacation/retirement treat to New Zealand and Australia. This past experience made Paul aware that he was of more use to his family taking care of the family home and keeping things in order than waiting in a hospital in Victoria for news of how Michelle was doing.

Paul loved serving others. And he knew he was doing his job. He felt needed and useful in the family's emergency plan. But he felt disconnected and alone, and being alone was something he had never liked and would normally try to avoid. It gave him too much time to think. This was a great challenge for Paul, although in retrospect, he felt it had given him some "awesome skills and perspectives for dealing with challenges that happen in everyday life."

At the time, Paul's girlfriend, Jenn, had been on a tour of Asia with the University of Victoria Chamber Choir. On the weekend of her return to Canada, a few days after Michelle's incident, Paul travelled to Vancouver and met Jenn and her parents at the airport. It was a surreal greeting for Paul, mixed with happiness and anxiety. Jenn's family dropped Paul off at the ferry where he walked on and continued his journey to Victoria to see Michelle.

When he saw Michelle in the hospital it was melancholy experience for Paul. Michelle seemed peaceful and relaxed, and there was an eerie serenity with the monotony of the machines whirring away keeping her breathing. Michelle was in a coma at the time. Being her little brother, Paul tried to keep a light hearted theme to his visits. He would tease her and speak in a Darth Vader voice. But it was an emotional time for Paul. Sometimes he would simply sit quietly and hold her hand. Once in a while he would find himself sniffling as a tear made its way down his face.

From time to time Paul would allow the unthinkable enter his mind; Michelle could die. But as her condition stabilized and she became conscious, his fears subsided. He couldn't help but worry, though, about her future. Michelle was so vibrant, so full of life. What would be her quality of life? Paul could only hope.

It wasn't difficult for Paul to visit his sister in the hospital. Unlike Michelle, who absolutely detested hospitals, he had no problem with a healthcare institution. His biggest problem was mustering up the energy to travel all the way across town from the University of Victoria to VGH. He would spend time working on the jigsaw puzzle that family and friends tackled together. In those first days and weeks many people came by to pay their respects. Paul dealt with it all in the best way he knew how, all the while feeling an overwhelming sense of helplessness. There was absolutely nothing he could do for his sister.

• • •

Michelle could recall an interesting relationship with her brother. "I remember when Paul was just a baby. He had quite a bit of hair and we girls went with Dad to buy a baby brush. He was always my cute little brother."

Michelle sometimes played Lego with Paul, or played in the sandbox. When Paul was just a baby, the Brittons bought a lake property. Michelle thought Paul always liked the lake. He would spend many hours snorkelling around the rocks.

It was Cori and Michelle who encouraged Paul to play football in high school. "He was always chubby so we thought sport might help," Cori explained. "Of course this meant going to an occasional game, even if it was cold or rainy."

When Michelle graduated, she, her parents, and Paul went to Europe. Cori couldn't go because she was working. Michelle and Paul had a great time. "Paul was my little buddy," she said of the trip. "We shared bunk-beds and jokes. Dad and Paul did some things together like climbing the stairs up Cathedral Steeple in Koln, Germany."

In the Victoria townhouse where Michelle lived with her brother, sister, and friend, Tammi, Michelle recalls that all of the roommates supported the importance of having dinner together every Sunday. This would always include Paul.

At that time, Paul drove their grandmother's old Valiant and he often let Michelle borrow it. Occasionally, she drove the car to work at the Oak Bay recreation center. But most often Paul let her take the car out to the airport where she took her flight training course.

There was one time Michelle remembers when "Paul surprised me as my guard dog. My boyfriend lived next door and one night in a drunken spurt of energy my boyfriend climbed over from their balcony to ours. Each town house had a connecting balcony with a board partitioning each. Bruce made so much noise he woke Paul, whose bedroom was between mine and the other townhouse. My room had the door and I let Bruce in. Well, Paul came in and tore a strip off him and kicked him out. It was funny later."

In the days, weeks, and months to come, Paul and Michelle would develop a truly unique brother and sister relationship. Evidence of his love for her would be shown in so many ways.

Chapter 7

It was a small, stark white room. The walls were bare. At one end, it appeared there was an explosion or something that had blasted a hole in the wall. There was a lot of destruction, but no smoke. It didn't look like a safe exit, but it was the only way out. Michelle thought she was in a hospital. No. Maybe it was a hotel. Yes, it would be better if it was a hotel. She really hated hospitals. She made her way across the damaged debris and through the wall that led to a narrow, dimly lit tunnel. The tunnel went on endlessly. There were other people around, passing by her, but nobody Michelle knew. Occasionally there was a pile of boxes stacked here and there throughout the tunnel. Some were piled higher than her head and she had to maneuver herself around them. It was a struggle doing this as the tunnel was only about three feet wide. The ceiling was maybe only 6 feet high. She tried not to panic. The tunnel seemed infinitely long.

Michelle's brain was working. Michelle was dreaming.

• • •

When Michelle was transferred to ICU in VGH she was kept in an enclosed environment as a precaution. Doctors suspected she may have meningitis. Friends and family were only allowed to visit her in the isolation room one at a time. Dr. Martin was the neurosurgeon in charge of Michelle's care. Dr. Waters handled Michelle's respiratory functions. So far, Michelle's condition remained a mystery.

CAT scans revealed no information. Even the spinal tap showed nothing out of the ordinary. Anne, one of the nurses, explained to the family what treatment Michelle was receiving. They had given Michelle small amounts of morphine along with muscle relaxants. Michelle's stomach was passing bile and some blood in her gastric tube, therefore, she had been given medication to settle her stomach.

The following morning, when the family returned very early to the hospital, they were told by Judy, the day nurse, that an E.E.G. had been done on Michelle and this test showed everything was fine. Michelle's thought processes appeared to be intact. They knew she could see and hear. And they knew she was aware. Of course, Michelle wasn't talking, because she had an airway tube taped to her mouth. The family would try to communicate with her, asking her to respond to questions with one blink of the eyes for 'yes' and two blinks for 'no.' But this seemed too difficult for Michelle. Then they tried having her simply open her eyes for 'yes.' They thought she was trying, but they didn't know for certain.

An MRI was scheduled for 3 pm that afternoon. Cori picked up Paul at the ferry and they visited Michelle in the ICU. Then Paul drove off to Vancouver to pick up his girlfriend, Jenn. A few hours later Dr. Martin spoke to the family, giving his thoughts on the results of the test. He suggested there was some indication of inflammation of the brain stem or possibly blood clots. He mentioned he may know more after consulting with the radiologist.

The family returned to the townhouse for dinner, and later went back to the hospital. Things were quiet. The nurses had changed shifts. Michelle rested. At about 10:30 that evening another neurologist, Dr. Kemble, examined Michelle. There was another test he wanted done, an arteriogram. The following day they all went back to the hospital. Hospital staff was working on some physiotherapy for Michelle's arms and legs. Michelle was booked for the arteriogram at 1:30, but it was cancelled. Dr. Martin explained to the family about the dangers involved with the test. Having shared these concerns, it was agreed that the arteriogram was definitely needed, despite the risk. Dr. Martin rebooked the test for 4 pm.

• • •

Then finally, a diagnosis. Spontaneous Arterial Dissection. The explanation from the doctors was complicated. The test showed a dissection of the right posterior ventricle artery in the brain stem. A dissection is a hole in the inner lining of the artery, causing blood to seep into the space between, pushing the lining of the artery inward to cause partial closure. In Michelle's case, this dissection created two small blood clots further down the arteries. In simple layperson's terms, it was a stroke. Doctors immediately gave Michelle the drug Heparin which is a blood thinner that helps prevent further blood clotting and would decrease the 'bubble' blocking one of the main arteries to Michelle's brain.

For the family, the meetings with doctors were ceaseless. Exhausting. They were asked the same questions over and over. Did Michelle ever see a chiropractor? Had Michelle experienced a recent fall? Was Michelle involved in any activities that would cause jarring of the body? Cori liked speaking with the neurosurgeon, Dr. Martin. He was trying to figure out why this had happened to Michelle. But Cori did not like the meetings with the other doctors. None of them were optimistic. These doctors told the family Michelle may never again get out of bed. She may never again breathe on her own. Nothing positive. And Cori felt sickened by Michelle being laid up in the ICU. There were tubes everywhere. It seemed more permanent. Michelle had now been sedated and was sleeping. Cori didn't like that. For Cori, the reality of Michelle's bleak situation was "starting to be so real and sink in." Cori didn't like that either, remembering, "I think I accepted all the doctors told us, at least about what had happened to her medically. But I didn't accept the prognosis, the future ideas they had about how she would or wouldn't get better. For doctors, they had to give us the usual 'we don't think she will ever get out of bed or talk again. I didn't believe that at all. Not my Michelle, feisty fighter that she is; with that stubborn 'do her own thing' type of attitude, she just wouldn't give in like they said."

• • •

Michelle had led a very busy life throughout her late teens and early twenties. She loved to travel, exploring Europe and Mexico and cruising up to Alaska. Other places she visited were Disneyland, Oregon, Nova Scotia, and Hawaii. Her favorite places, Australia, New Zealand, and Fiji, she had travelled to twice.

On Michelle's very first solo trip she ventured to Australia and stayed a week with family friends in Sydney. Michelle felt she had led a pretty sheltered life up until then. She didn't feel she was experienced at being self-sufficient. For example, she wasn't even accustomed to using the phone book. Consequently, she initially felt lost and overwhelmed. She didn't know what to do with herself. There, she was completely free to do whatever she wanted; there was no one but Michelle herself to decide her route or means of travel. It was both exhilarating and unnerving.

Michelle's adventurous spirit led her to trying all sorts of new things. While working in Banff she attempted rock climbing. Her climb was only about sixty feet, yet, she felt a tingle of excitement with hearing the howling wind. And she was invigorated by the little rush of adrenaline. While in Banff there were lots of activities including hiking, roller blading, and mountain biking.

In Australia, she loved her plane ride in a little Cessna 205 that took off and landed on the beach, something Michelle knew would never happen in Canada. In New Zealand she tried splunking and black water rafting. Spelunking, or caving, was where she and some friends donned wet suits and head lamps and floated on a tube through the caves. To Michelle, "it was cold, wet, and dark, but very worth it". She also took her turn on a zip line that ran across a ravine. She went horse trekking. This was no "slow trot through the woods" but an excursion up a rolling hill and through the fields. Sometimes the guide would allow the more experienced riders to gallop ahead and wait for the others at the next fence. Luckily Michelle was capable on a horse and she was not afraid to take off for a good run.

Michelle also went skydiving. It was tandem, so she didn't need much instruction. On the jump she was so afraid she closed her eyes, but the instructor yelled at her to keep her eyes open and take in the view. And there were so many hiking adventures. One memorable hike was through fields and fields of sheep under a star filled night sky. This was near Mount Cook.

When Michelle was in Fiji she ventured under water for some scuba diving near a reef, marveling at the brilliant colors of the coral, fish, and sea animals. On her second trip to Fiji she tried parasailing and thought it was great. She even chanced a swim from one island to another. It didn't seem too far, and the water was warm. She and her English companion made it to the other island, though the return trip seemed to take forever and she felt very relieved to finally feel the sand beneath her feet.

In New Zealand, Michelle boogie boarded down the sand dunes near the beach. She also went sea kayaking and sailing. She thought the sea kayaking was "brilliant," paddling in the open ocean for a while, then up an estuary to a waterfall. She and a youth hostel companion, an Irish girl, sailed with a couple from Scotland and a German fellow. They sailed on a 40 foot yacht called *She's A Lady*. Each of the novice sailors took a turn at the wheel. Another adventure Michelle tried was white water sledging. These risk takers would paddle down the river wearing wet suits, and float on their stomachs on a foam sled. Michelle loved the thrill of being tossed around on the chilly white water waves. She gave surfing a try with a group of friends in Cairns. She found surfing quite difficult and knew she didn't do well at it, but still she had fun. On a stay at a horse ranch, along with developing a special interaction with her horse, Michelle also learned how to throw a boomerang.

• • •

So this was the active, adventurous young woman who had been suddenly stricken down to a fragile girl, lying in a hospital bed, tubes running into her near lifeless body. It was a tragic event that stunned those who knew her; loved her. Dr. Martin said he would never in a month of Sundays have expected that a 24 year old would suffer a stroke in the brain stem area. That was why he had asked so many questions about Michelle's activities and experiences in the days and weeks before she ended up in the hospital. A stroke in the brain stem was a very rare occurrence. Doctor Martin had only seen such a devastating injury four times in his career of thirty odd years. Cases of this type of incident may have been only 150 in the whole world.

Was it Michelle's active lifestyle that led to this damage? Was Michelle's neck twisted too hard one night when she fell on the dance floor at a local bar? Was something jarred when she jumped on her cousin's trampoline? Did that small whiplash she received begin the rupture of her vein? Nobody had a clear answer. This was a mystery that would never be solved.

• • •

The news of Michelle's diagnosis was heartbreaking for Sandy Fulton, the social worker. She recalls:

"As a health care provider in a team of health care professionals you know what outcomes can be. You know if this person doesn't recover what the quality of their life is going to be like.

And so do you encourage the family to say enough is enough? Let's stop? Or you don't encourage the family to do that, you encourage the family to make their own decisions. You have to let them know what it can be like and that's my role I believe I practice as a social worker, without damning people to hell, but you have to have the information. Some would say, 'Are you kidding me!' Again, you just don't come right out and blatantly say this is what I think. Physicians will say that. And they're doing that based on what they know. The other piece is, you don't take away hope. If you take away hope, what the hell is there? You can't take away hope. I must say the Intensivists here in the intensive care unit for the most part are extremely kind. They're very good at patient conferences. A lot of people don't come out of ICU. They are there because they are not going to get better. The ICU staff always appreciates it when somebody comes back and says, 'Remember me?'"

• • •

A report from the Occupational Therapy Department included detailed information about Michelle's past life. Interviews with the family gave therapists information about where Michelle had been living, who she was living with, that she had just completed her Bachelor of Commerce Degree, specializing in tourism. Therapists knew that Michelle had travelled extensively. They mentioned New Zealand, Australia and Fiji in their reports. It was written that Michelle enjoyed an active lifestyle including running and cycling, and that she was working towards her pilot's license.

The report noted that Michelle was in a "total care" condition. She had no spontaneous movements except for her eyes. Her mental status was still unknown. Michelle was closing her eyes "possibly to decrease stimulation." At a caregiver support group meeting various concerns were addressed. The therapist indicated that Michelle did not have a consistent method of communication. It was also noted that she had far too much stimulation in her environment. This was something that was not the best thing for a person dealing with major brain trauma. Quiet surroundings would calm her nerves.

The plan was to work with Michelle, encouraging her to respond to one step commands that only required her to do one thing at a time. All those involved with her were to tone down the noise and other stimulating activities, limiting visitors to two at a time. All who visited with her were encouraged to document daily events in her diary. The occupational therapist would consider various communication options.

• • •

Michelle was in a cabin room of a large cruise ship. The ship was docked. She could see through the window. There was land all around. A rock wall towered outside. People were climbing upwards. Michelle watched.

Even in her dreams Michelle's mind led her towards adventure.

Chapter 8

Tammi Henderson had made her decision to pursue a career in hotel management. She enrolled in the University College of the Caribou (UCC). That was where she would meet Michelle, as both young women were enrolled in the Resort Hotel Management program. This program involved two years of studying at the university along with working for a while at a participating hotel. After the first round of school studies was completed, students were required to move on to the practicum at the hotel. The girls finished their first part of the program in May and Tammi, Michelle, and another older girl, Tania, moved to Banff to work at the Rimrock Hotel. Students from the hotel management course were of all ages, Tania being a couple of years older than Michelle and Tammi. Consequently, it was Tammi and Michelle, both around the same age, who started a friendship that would grow into a special and everlasting bond.

Staff accommodations at the Rimrock were in the bottom of the hotel. It was one huge room with 3 separate beds, along with one bathroom they all shared. Each girl had her own little fridge. Michelle and Tammi were the very first female dishwashers in this hotel, surrounded by lots of guys who were very excited to see girl's names on the work schedule. Tammi was to soon find out that sharing the hotel with lots of men was a perfect situation for Michelle. Michelle, in Tammi's eyes, was definitely a 'boy girl,' meaning "there are some girls that just get along better with men and that's just the way it is, and she's definitely like that for sure."

Tammi and Michelle spent the summer "just dishwashing and having a good time and getting to know each other." They hiked together all around the Banff area, although Tammi was too scared to join Michelle in her adventurous rock climbing. Tammi liked the outgoing part of Michelle's personality. She found her new friend easy to talk to. Michelle would "let you talk and then give you advice." If Michelle thought there was something Tammi could do to make a situation better, then Michelle would make suggestions of things she could try.

The way things worked out, Tammi returned to Kamloops to write a test at UCC while Michelle stayed on a little longer in Banff. The two girls then continued finishing up their hotel management course together in Kamloops. After their course was completed, Tammi received a phone call from the Rimrock Hotel and was asked if she would come back and manage one of the hotel's departments. So Tammi went back to Banff. And Michelle went to Australia. Tammi worked in Banff for two years while Michelle spent the summer in Australia and then moved out to Victoria to be with her sister. Michelle had enrolled in her two year degree program at the university there. The girls kept in close touch with each other through phone calls, emails, and also letters. Michelle, a couple of times, ventured up to Banff for a visit. And the two young women were always home in Kamloops at the same time during spring breaks and Christmas.

After two years of working in Banff, Tammi was getting to that age in her life where she didn't want to do it anymore. She wanted a career. She felt that Banff was just a transient town, a party town, and it seemed that partying was all she did. Tammi mentioned this to Michelle one time when they were talking on the phone and Michelle said, "Well, why don't you move to Victoria?" Michelle's sister, Cori, who had been teaching English in Korea, was moving back to Canada. And their brother was also planning to move to Victoria. They had been talking about all of them renting a condo together. Tammi was hesitant. She didn't want to encroach on the family's plans. She told Michelle she liked the idea of moving to Victoria but wanted the approval of Michelle's siblings. But Michelle was insistent, and Tammi soon joined the Britton gang. It was only some time later, after Tammi had blended happily with all three siblings, that Michelle confessed to Tammi Cori's problem with the whole plan. Cori was not happy about Tammi moving in with them. Cori did not know Tammi and really did not want Tammi living with them. But Michelle had told her sister, "Well, it's going to happen." And everything was fine. Tammi wound up being really good friends with both Cori and Paul. Nowadays, when Cori travels from her home in Calgary to visit family in Kamloops, she always phones Tammi.

• • •

Within two weeks of moving to Victoria, having her Resort Hotel Management degree in hand, Tammi landed a job as a server at the Empress Hotel. This was where Tammi was working when she received the life-changing call from Cori. It was a confusing call. Cori was upset and crying, it was difficult to understand what she was talking about. Cori couldn't say exactly what had happened. She mentioned Michelle being in the hospital and wanted Tammi to come to the hospital right away. Tammi asked what was going on but Cori could not give her any details. She just wanted Tammi to get there, fast.

Tammi hung up the phone. She had been right in the middle of getting a lunch taken down, but she dropped everything. She was now in a panic. She ran out of the kitchen into a back area. Her manager chased after her and asked her what was wrong. Tammi could not explain. She blurted out "I have to go. I can't be here. I have to go to the hospital." Staff gathered around a totally distraught Tammi. They calmed her down. She tried to explain to them what was happening. But she didn't know much herself. She just wanted to go.

So Tammi got in her car and drove, and ended up at the hospital in the emergency area. She found Cori there, crying. She embraced her, holding her close until she calmed. They were right beside the emergency area and could just go in there where Michelle was. There was a bunch of people laid up. Michelle was there with a curtain pulled around her bed. Tammi had never before witnessed someone in an emergency ward. Her best friend was flat on her back, comatose, with tubes all over. Michelle was sleeping, just sleeping.

Tammi held Michelle's hand. It was so hard seeing her this way. It was agonizing not knowing what was going on. A nurse came by and started taking blood from Michelle. Tammi was a bit shocked and stunned. The nurse noticed this and said, "Oh, you're not a needle person. Then you'll have to leave the room." Tammi protested that there was no way she would leave that room. The nurse quite bluntly said, "Well, if you're going to pass out I need you to leave because we have to look after *her*." Tammi replied that she would just turn her head, because she wasn't going anywhere. She was determined to remain with her friend.

And it was good that Tammi was there. Cori was busy with the doctors, all of them trying to figure out what was happening with Michelle. For a long time Tammi stood by Michelle's bedside, holding her hand. Hours passed by, and many tests were done. Eventually the doctors made the decision to transfer Michelle to the other hospital. Hospital staff told the girls to go home for a while. The nurses needed time to prepare Michelle for the move. Cori and Tammi went home to their townhouse and refreshed themselves, changed their clothes. Tammi didn't once think of Michelle dying. She and Cori were so puzzled by the mystery of Michelle's sudden illness. The girls didn't know anything. The doctors didn't know anything. It was a major concern.

Later on in the day, at VGH, Cori and Tammi began the long wait at the ICU. Tammi remembers Michelle being comatose for about four hours. This was such a new experience for Tammi. She really didn't know what to do in the hospital, somewhat afraid she would do something wrong. But then, she didn't care so much about that, because the person who was lying there was a person who was very important to Tammi. Her main concern was to take care of Michelle. Tammi's co-workers had actually shown up at the hospital before she and Cori arrived. They all knew Michelle, and were there to offer their support. Tammi thought that was nice. One at a time they visited with Michelle. Doctors insisted that visits be short. Everyone understood that. When Tammi went in to see her, Michelle's eyes were open, but Tammi could tell Michelle was confused about what was happening to her. And Michelle couldn't talk. It was awful.

Eventually, Tammi went back to work and finished off her day. When she went back to the hospital, Michelle's parents had arrived. It was so emotional. Michelle's mom seemed to be the strong one. Michelle's dad seemed to stand back, sort of reserved. It seemed to Tammi that he just didn't know what to do at the moment. She could tell that the lack of answers from the doctors was very frustrating for both of Michelle's parents, as it was for everyone.

For Tammi, this was the beginning of a test of true friendship.

• • •

Dr. Kemble was asked to give a second opinion on Michelle's condition. He concluded that "Michelle presents with 'locked in' syndrome."

Chapter 9

Scott was the love of her life. Michelle met him through Cori while he was stationed in Victoria with the Navy. They had such a good time together and became incredibly close. His personality was larger than life; he was very social and outgoing, a lot of fun, very much alive. Everything was worth exploring. They spent many evenings at the Crossroads country bar. Michelle was quite a drinker and, in those days, beer was her choice of beverage. They drank beer and learned several different dance steps, including the swing and the two-step. It was such a great time they had dancing together. They laughed and laughed. Scott made everything fun.

Both Michelle and Scott were enrolled in flight training at the same school. Scott was ahead of Michelle with his flying and already had his private pilot license. Because he was working on his commercial pilot license, he was required to plan and take lots of flights to accumulate hours of flying. Of course, Michelle would accompany him on many of these trips.

One time they flew up Vancouver Island from Victoria to Campbell River, a small place, kind of a fishing town. Then they took off across the island to Long Beach where they spent the day relaxing in the sun. On another trip they flew down the Oregon coast to North Bend. They stopped at Friday harbor for a customs check and landed at another place for gas. Michelle wasn't thrilled with North Bend, as it was just another little town, but Scott wanted to make the most of it. He took Michelle for some wine tasting, then they Christmas shopped. Later on they briefly checked out the local casino.

One especially exciting time for Michelle was when Scott sneaked her onto his navy base after the 11 o'clock curfew. She curled up inside the trunk of his car. It was very dark, but she could hear everything. It was a bit naughty and a whole lot of fun. Scott probably could have gotten into trouble; however, Michelle stayed overnight and left unnoticed the next day. Their clandestine operation had been successful.

One of the absolute best experiences of their adventures was when they flew at night over the spectacular city of Vancouver. The experience made both of them feel the freedom of a soaring Peter Pan. On the days when they were not exploring the skies, Scott would visit Michelle at her place, sometimes showing up with a bottle of wine, usually red. They would eat noodle soup and watch a movie.

The happy couple dated for about nine months. The premise was for them to keep their relationship on a casual basis. Well, that didn't happen. Michelle was very much in love with this guy, and could envision spending the rest of her life with him. They often talked of their future plans. Scott wanted to join the Air Force and move back to Nova Scotia. Michelle desired to finish getting her pilot's license, and would then learn to fly helicopters.

But unfortunately the relationship turned into a bit of a chore for Scott. Michelle could sense something was wrong. There was about a week of "crazy bad vibes" between them. There were too many awkward silences. For Scott, it was time to move on. It was not in his plan to marry, and he told Michelle exactly that: he would never marry her. He was ready to transfer to the Air Force and move back home to Nova Scotia. Maybe he and Michelle could have shared a lifetime together had they met a little later on in their lives, when Scott was more settled in his career and ready for a permanent relationship. But it was not meant to be. Scott broke things off with Michelle and she was devastated. She contacted Scott a few times after the breakup and pleaded to get back together, but he had made up his mind. Michelle cried steadily for a week, feeling totally abandoned. She was really quite a mess. But, even though she was heartbroken, her friendship with Scott survived the romance and they would still see each other from time to time.

As time passed, Scott did transfer to the Air Force, and he did move back to Nova Scotia. Michelle had actually been to the east coast of Canada, the Maritime Provinces, when she was much younger. She had travelled there with her parents. She decided she would go there again and visit Scott. She convinced him over the phone to allow her to see him. He agreed to let her come to his place, but was very clear at that time that it was to be strictly platonic between them.

So, two months after her breakup with Scott, Michelle travelled to Nova Scotia. She met him at the Halifax airport. It was so good to see him. The weather that day was overcast and drizzling rain. They retrieved Michelle's bag and Scott drove her to his new house close to the military base. It was a simple two story house with a big flat back yard. Scott gave her a tour of the place. He basically lived on the top floor. His bedroom was at one end, and a hallway led to a bedroom at the other end. Along the hall were a den and a bathroom. Off the same hall was an open living room and kitchen with bright yellow flowery wall paper.

Scott still had a couple of days of work before he took a break, so Michelle entertained herself running each morning and checking out the local area. The terrain was flat, the surroundings rural. On Friday night she and Scott went to the bar for a while. They had a couple beers and danced. They definitely knew how move well together.

The next day they packed up and drove to his parent's place in Halifax. Scott's parents lived in a very comfortable home and Michelle was happy to see them. She had previously met Scott's dad when he visited Vancouver Island, but this was the first time she met his mom.

Their travels around Nova Scotia would take a counter-clockwise route. Michelle was very impressed with how pretty this province was and took lots of pictures. Tourist season had not yet begun as it was only April. This meant that staying in hotels was quite cheap and Scott could also get a military discount. They slept together in the same bed, but there was no physical romantic involvement. Scott held true to his need to keep their relationship on a strictly friendship level. Michelle was disappointed, yet she knew him well enough to know he was a man who stood by his word.

In Yarmouth the two of them visited with some of Scott's friends and had a few drinks. They drove up north and had dinner at an old English style pub. As they drove further in the northern area, Michelle noticed this weird green light through the back window. Scott told her it was the Northern Lights. Michelle had seen these lights a few times in Kamloops, but never like this. Here in Nova Scotia, the lights were so bright and so green. It was marvelous.

Through their drive around Cape Breton Scott was feeling a little under the weather, so Michelle drove while he slept. Later on they spent some time exploring the rocks around Peggy's cove. Having completed the circle tour, they went back to spend some more time at his parent's place. Scott's parents did most of their living in the downstairs area of the house. In the main recreation room were a wood stove, a bar, and a television. Scott's dad had a den down the hall where he had his computer and short wave radio. During her stay there Michelle also met Scott's grandmother and his older brother. And of course there was the family dog, Skip.

One evening Michelle and Scott went downtown to the bars. There were a few different bars that they walked through, and they ran into a few of Scott's friends. Michelle was a very social young woman and loved meeting all of these people. She was especially impressed with the guy who worked on a submarine. Later on she and Scott ventured into an old tavern with a very low ceiling. The place was packed. They stayed long enough to listen to a folk singer perform a couple of maritime songs. Michelle loved this part of the culture.

Then, all too quickly, the vacation was over and it was time for Michelle to go back home. Deep down she had wished something romantic would happen between her and Scott. There had been that hope he might still feel something for her. But it didn't happen. And Michelle realized that it was never going to happen, that this episode of her life was over. Scott could no longer be in that special place in her heart.

• • •

Scott Guthrie had a slightly different interpretation of the relationship between himself and Michelle.

He was working as a Steward in the Canadian Navy. He was also working as the bar manager of the Pacific Fleet Club in Victoria, BC. During this time he was also attending Victoria Flight Training, taking his private pilot's license and moving towards a career in commercial aviation.

Scott and Cori met through mutual friends while both were living in Victoria. The two of them became very good friends and partied together every weekend for an entire summer. It became customary for Scott to crash at Cori's apartment after a night of fun downtown. Their relationship was never anything more than friends.

Then one day, Michelle returned from Australia and moved in with her sister. Scott continued to hang out and crash at their place on the weekends and, in Scott's words, "Michelle and I became more than just friends." When Scott first met Michelle he was taken aback by how beautiful she was, not just her physical beauty, but "her sheer beauty of existence." She was always exuberant and cheerful. She possessed a wonderful sense of humor. She exhumed kindness and was so easy to talk to. "Not to mention those eyes... those eyes that can light up the darkest corners of the deepest abyss and turn it into a glistening sapphire sanctuary of happiness."

The relationship between Scott and Michelle "just kind of happened." They hung out on weekends, Scott crashing at their apartment, and they would often wind up innocently cuddling up watching TV, drinking wine and falling asleep. It felt so good to be together. Their innocent cuddles and friendship quickly turned into something more intimate and they soon found themselves spending more and more time with each other.

The young lovers had many memorable times together. Once or twice a week they would go to the country bar downtown on Discovery Street to learn some country dancing. It was at this bar that they met Roberta, another good friend of both Michelle and Scott. Roberta even became Scott's roommate for a while.

One of the best trips of Scott's life was the time when he and Michelle went on a long flight together. Part of Scott's commercial rating with his pilot training was his requirement to do a 500 kilometer cross country trip. He and Michelle talked about it and studied some maps. They decided that North Bend, Oregon would be an interesting trip. The two of them jumped into a Cessna 172 and made the trip on a weekend. On the way south they took an inland route via Seattle. They made a couple of stops along the way for fuel and made it to North Bend without incident. They spent a night at a hotel and then flew back up north along the West Coast for the return trip. It was beautiful, looking over the ocean and the mountains at the same time. During that trip Scott felt he and Michelle grew quite close. "Spending that much time together in a small aircraft certainly gives you lots of time to talk to each other."

Scott recalls they were together for about nine months. It was a combination of things that eventually caused their breakup. Scott was certainly not ready to settle down. Most of his reluctance to commit to a long term relationship, he felt, stemmed back to his childhood. When Scott was young his father was in the Navy. Scott never really knew his father very well in those years. His dad would go away for six months at a time, come home for a short while and then disappear again. Scott never really understood "why he was never there for us." As kids, Scott and his brother would live their lives under their mother's rules for long periods of time. Then, "like a flick of a switch my dad would come home and everything would change, usually for the worse." Scott never had anyone to teach him how to hold a baseball bat, catch a ball, or hold a hockey stick. He and his brother very rarely had their dad around to teach them much of anything. All Scott could remember as a child was that the "rules would change and my parents would fight." Scott swore he would never subject his children to such a thing as they grew up. And that was why Scott held off settling down with anyone, for fear it would lead to having children that would never see him.

The actual timing of Scott's and Michelle's breakup was closely linked to Scott's posting out of Victoria. He accepted an occupational transfer out of the Navy into the Air Force as an Aviations Systems Technician (basically an Aircraft Mechanic). He was posted to Borden, Ontario for training for over a year. His training at Aviation School was to be followed by a posting to anywhere in Canada. Michelle was still finishing her University degree and they knew they would not see each other for quite some time. They spoke about options and where their relationship was heading. They agreed that it would be best if they took a break from their relationship so they could focus on their schooling and see where they both were after school. However, Scott suspected the breakup was more his wish than Michelle's.

During their time apart Scott thought of Michelle often and they kept in touch. When Scott completed his training, he and Michelle decided she should come and visit him in his new home in

Greenwood, Nova Scotia, where he finally ended up being posted with the Air Force. About Michelle's visit, he recalls,

"Wow, what a great visit. I picked her up at the airport and we spent the first night at my house. Over the next number of days, we embarked on a whirl wind tour of Nova Scotia. We visited The Annapolis Valley, Digby, Yarmouth, the South Shore, Halifax, Truro, Pictou, Antigonish, Cape Breton Highland, the Eastern Shore, and then back to Halifax. I remember it was a lot of ground to cover in such a short time. It was a great time, taking lots of pictures and laughing a lot. A part of me was thinking that she may return (to Nova Scotia) after her University to live, and things could move on from there."

• • •

It was a phone call Scott remembered well. Cori was the one who had called him. Scott was on vacation at his family cottage on Prince Edward Island with a couple of friends. The week had been busy and he'd just spent a long day working around the property. In the very early hours of the morning, about 2 or 3 am, Scott's cell phone began to ring. This in itself was very strange. The cottage was located in an area with very poor cellular reception. Whenever Scott would use his phone "usually you'd need to be outside standing at just the right place, at the right angle to even get a signal and even then it is awful." Oddly, the reception on that night was crystal clear. Cori delivered the bad news and asked if he would come. Scott was shocked and spent the rest of the late hours trying to figure out what to do. As soon as the sun rose, he woke his guests and told them to pack their bags. He would drop them off at a train station in Truro, Nova Scotia so they could continue their vacation. By about 10 am the same day, Scott had returned home to Greenwood and went straight to his workplace to request an extended vacation so he could go out west. After a brief explanation of what had happened, Scott received the time off.

At this point in his career, Scott was working for 434 Combat Support Squadron. The squadron flew T-33 Silverstar Aircraft (T-Bird) and CT-144 Challenger Jets. The Challenger is a small business class jet that the military had converted to carry out various electronic warfare roles as well as fulfill a role in medical evacuation.

For the average person, a plan to travel from coast to coast in Canada would take several days. But for Scott, with fate being on his side, he was in the air within hours.

He had been standing by the operations desk explaining his situation to some co-workers, telling them how he was anxiously trying to find his way back to Michelle. A pilot was standing close by and interrupted the conversation. The pilot explained that he was actually departing in one hour to go do operations on the West Coast out of Comox, BC. The pilot suggested that if Scott could be sitting on the aircraft ready to go within an hour, he would have a ride to BC.

After a quick chat with his Commanding Officer, finishing some paperwork, and a lightning quick dash home to get some things, Scott returned to the base, hopped on the aircraft and was on his way. It was early afternoon when the plane took off. It made a brief stop for about an hour in Cold Lake, Alberta, and flew on to Comox.

Scott was terrified and feared for the worst. He did not know what was going to happen, but he certainly thought Michelle's death was a possibility and "it scared the living crap out of me." The night before, in the wee hours of the morning, he had not been able to sleep. His head was swimming with possibilities and he was not sure if he was going to make it to see Michelle before she passed away. Not knowing what had happened to her or why was "just horrible." At the time when he was packing his bags, getting ready to leave the cottage, all he could think was "I have to see her, I have to help her, I have to do something."

When the plane landed in Comox, there was a car waiting for Scott to drive him to Victoria. It had been less than 24 hours from the time of that late night phone call to the moment Scott was standing on Cori's doorstep. He spent most of the night talking with Cori and her family.

Scott was worn out. He needed some sleep. But his concern for Michelle consumed his mind. Even though he and Michelle had actually ended their relationship, this did not change how he felt for her. The two of them had shared many intimate moments together. Scott had fallen in love with her and was still deeply captivated by "who she is." And, even though he tried to deny his feelings to justify staying single, his profound love for her was still there. And sleep would not come.

The following morning they all went into the hospital to see Michelle. It was a very emotional time. Lots of tears, lots of unknowns. They were not sure if she would wake up or survive "or what the hell was going on in her head." To see her lying there, virtually helpless, on life support "darned near floored me." To Scott, she certainly did not look like Michelle. Although he knew it was her, it was only her shell. Everything "that makes her who she is was missing." Her smile, her laugh, her humor, her attitude, her voice; all of who she was, all missing. This scared Scott and he wanted to burst out and cry. There were lots of tears that day. So many tears.

• • •

It was Scott who purchased the daily diary that would be kept at Michelle's bedside throughout her ordeal at VGH. The diary was a wonderful idea, yet Scott added even more to this detailed account. He flipped through the pages and wrote cute little messages to Michelle; usually he doodled a goofy face. He picked out days of special events throughout the calendar, days that would matter to Michelle. Not knowing how long she would stay in the hospital, and knowing he could not be there with her, he wrote something on every special occasion for the full year. He left a Happy Birthday note in May. In June he wrote on the top of one page, "205 Days Til X-mas." Later in that month he left a note asking the family if they had called him today. He signed it with love.

At the end of July Scott wrote in the diary, sending Michelle a big hug from across the country. His drawing of his goofy guy had outstretched arms. In the August section he mentioned only 117 days until Christmas and hoped that she was feeling better. In December he wrote, "Have you got all your Christmas shopping done? Don't forget about me!!!" On December 25 he wrote out "Merry Christmas Shelly, Love, Scott" in artistic bold lettering. He drew a tiny mistletoe picture and a large goofy face donning a Santa hat. He drew a little Rudolf reindeer head with the caption, "Rudolf Loves You Too."

On December 31, Scott wrote, "Happy New Years, Michelle. Wish I could be there with you right now to bring it in with you. I love you and am thinking about you. Big Hugs and Kisses. Be good. Be strong. And don't let the day get to you. Lots of love with all of my heart. Scott."

The caption with his goofy face drawing read, "Keep Smiling."

Sandy Fulton did her best to help the Britton family deal with the stress and confusion involving Michelle's serious condition. For Joan and Gordon, Sandy organized a family conference.

Sandy comments, "Everybody hears the same thing at the same time. Cori hears it then tries to tell mom and dad. There might be something missed in translation, in terminology, all of those things. When mom and dad hear it they are at a different emotional place so they may not communicate that information effectively, so we like to have a family conference so that physician, nursing, social worker are present."

This was a customary procedure when patients were in ICU. The patients here were in a more intense situation than any other area in the hospital and careful communication with family was essential. Sandy knew it was very important to get a conference going "and making sure that everybody's questions are answered, that the physicians and nursing staff have the chance to say what it is that they need to say and that family don't walk away thinking, 'gee I didn't ask that' or 'what did that mean?'"

Chapter 10

In the first week Michelle had lots of visitors, her mom and dad and, of course, Cori. Her best friend, Tammi, was there every day. Grandma Britton came to the hospital and visited with her for an entire afternoon. Scott flew in from Nova Scotia and stayed a few days. Paul Newman came to see Michelle quite often. He was once the minister of the Kamloops United Church, and now lived on Vancouver Island. Kristy Broderick, a very good childhood friend of Michelle's, came to visit, though she almost fainted. Leanne, Jordon and Tannis came to see Michelle. They were co-workers with Tammi and knew Michelle quite well. They brought a basket of goodies.

The abundance of people surrounding Michelle was a bit disturbing to Cori. "I remember everyone would come and see Michelle, which is great, but I was used to having time by myself with her all the time (ever since we shared our room together when we were babies) and I was feeling like I wasn't getting 'my' time with my sister I loved so much. There were many things I shared with only her and I couldn't do that when others were there all the time. I was missing that."

• • •

Kristy Broderick and Michelle were both born in Kamloops, both born at the Royal Inland Hospital and both children of mothers named Joan. The girl's mothers were friends and took nursing training together. Kristy was actually closer to Cori in age, being almost two years older than Michelle. When Kristy was a toddler and preschooler she played mostly with Cori. Michelle played more with Kristy's younger brother, Kieran.

When Kristy was 6 years old her father accepted a job transfer and moved the family to Williams Lake. Kristy went to school there and graduated. But she still kept in touch with the Brittons. Her family visited Kamloops often and mainly stayed at the Britton home. Cori, Michelle and Kristy hung out during those visits. Kristy remembered Michelle as an easygoing young girl with a great sense of humor and a wonderful laugh.

After she completed high school, Kristy remained in Williams Lake and went to college for a year. She continued her education at the University of Victoria (UVic). During her first years of university, she lived in the UVic residence with Cori. Several years later Michelle went to Victoria and moved in with her sister. Kristy moved across town and began substitute teaching, and Michelle began working in the reservations department at one of the local hotels in downtown Victoria.

Cori left for about a year to work overseas teaching English. It was at this time that Michelle and Kristy began spending a lot of time together. They hung out with other friends and frequented the local pubs quite often. They also went to nightclubs or would go see a movie. Kristy liked Cori's little sister. "Michelle was always lots of fun, a positive person, and she had a contagious laugh. The guys we would meet were always attracted to Michelle's beautiful smile and her bubbly personality!"

It was a year or so later when Cori, Michelle, Paul, and Tammi moved in together near the University of Victoria. Kristy would still see Michelle from time to time, but Michelle was quite busy in those days with her Commerce courses at the university.

• • •

Kristy hadn't heard from Michelle for over a week, but didn't think much about it. Michelle was busy with schooling and her job. Cori phoned her and gave her the bad news: Michelle had suffered a stroke. Cori's voice seemed anxious as she filled Kristy in on what had happened, but she also seemed optimistic that her sister would be fine. Kristy was "very worried," however, she had no doubt Michelle would be okay. In Kristy's encounters with other family and friends who had experienced strokes, they had all gotten better over time. Kristy "truly thought it would be the same with Michelle and because she was young she would recover faster."

But when Kristy went to see Michelle the next day in ICU and spoke to Michelle's family, reality quickly dampened her hopes. This was not a common stroke. It was in a very rare area of the brain. It had affected Michelle's entire body. Kristy was devastated for Michelle, her family, and her friends.

Although Kristy wasn't family, she was allowed to go in to see Michelle in ICU. She was stunned at the sight of her friend. "Michelle was hooked up to monitors and tubes. It was then that I realized that what had happened to her was much worse than I had ever thought. Everything was very overwhelming…the monitors, the tubes, the nurses checking on her, etc. Here was this young, healthy, vivacious, beautiful, fun loving young lady lying lifeless in the bed." Kristy was devastated "beyond belief." She nearly passed out on that visit; "It was just too much to take in."

• • •

Michelle had long hair. It felt like someone was constantly pulling her ponytail, a slight tugging at the back of her head. It didn't hurt. It was just bothersome, not normal. She could not see well at all. Everything was fuzzy; people around her were merely shadows with faces she could not recognize. And there were lots and lots of people busily doing things with her. Every morning the lab nurse would take her blood. Michelle felt like a pin cushion. Unfortunately for Michelle, it was difficult for medical staff to find her veins. On average, it took four tries to insert the needle properly. One time they could only find a good vein in her right big toe.

Michelle could not move anything. Anything! She could not even turn her head. And, because she had a tube down her throat to make sure she was breathing and getting enough oxygen, she could not talk or even make a sound. Her sense of touch was completely gone. It was as if her body was simply not there from the neck down. Her brain and body went into survival mode. Mostly, she slept. When she was awake, her existence was confusing. She could only focus on the present moment. Every few hours nurses would suction fluid from her lungs. Four times a day she would be fed through a long tube with a bag on the end. The bag was attached to a "kangaroo pump" that would regulate the amount of food going into her stomach.

Michelle "just wasn't all there" for a long time. She was visited by rarely seen relatives from Vancouver, which made her suspect something really bad had happened to her. At this point the quality of her life did not exist. She really didn't care "about life or anything." She was mainly dealing with the mountain of medical stuff that was so new. Occasionally, a terrifying thought would come to her, "Is this my life now?"

• • •

Michelle's diagnosis was unbelievable. Cori was dazed and devastated. But she was also very determined. The horrible future doctors predicted for Michelle was not going to happen. Cori would help her. It was agonizing to think this all could have been prevented if Michelle had only seen a doctor when she'd first had the headaches. But when doctors informed the family that Michelle's persistent headaches would have only led them to believe they were migraines, this was very comforting to Cori. At most, doctors would have done a CAT scan and possibly an MRI, neither of which would have indicated that Michelle was headed towards such a traumatic event.

For Cori, there was never that stunning moment when Michelle dramatically revealed her cognitive abilities. Cori always knew that her sister could think clearly, or at least she hoped she did. Cori never thought otherwise. Those first few days and weeks in the hospital were a crazy dream to Cori. She recalls seeming to know intuitively, "twin-like", what Michelle wanted, when others around her could not figure it out. She cannot remember, though, how she and Michelle began communicating through the process of Michelle blinking her eyes. It seemed to come naturally. Cori sensed that Michelle was having trouble with blinking her eyes once for yes and twice for no. Michelle seemed to open her eyes wider for yes, and blink once for no. Cori understood this. There was encouraging progress with Michelle's condition. She was coughing fairly well. This was a hopeful sign that Michelle could one day breath on her own without the help of a ventilator. And maybe she would no longer have to be suctioned. Cori could tell that Michelle did not like the suctioning. On the fifth day in the hospital, Michelle developed bronchitis and was put on antibiotics.

Michelle's lips were swelling, probably from the tape that fastened her breathing tube to her mouth. Tammi was so upset by this. She felt so horrible for Michelle. She wanted to somehow deflate those puffy lips. She just wanted all those awful attachments removed. "Oh my God," she kept thinking. "Take them off!"

To Cori, the problem with Michelle's swollen lips was something she had not even noticed. Cori was "giving only positive thoughts to Michelle and talking about my day and talking to her about things the nurses had mentioned…I looked at her as if she were still the Michelle I always knew…I saw tubes, but they didn't bother me after a while; I guess I started to ignore them. I was really just into being with Michelle and giving her all my positive energy to heal well and get better."

Dr. Dyson from UVic Health Services arrived to see Michelle. Under the circumstances he felt Michelle should be given her degree without 'COOP.' A COOP was where students would take classes for 4 months then work for 4 months in a related field from which the student received credits. The student would then take 4 more months of classes and do another 4 months of working, and so on, until they had done this four times. Michelle had already completed four of her sessions of classes and three of her work requirements. She only had one 4 month work term to go. Dr. Dyson offered to speak on her behalf to the Dean of UVic. It was a nice gesture.

Spending time at the hospital with Michelle soon became part of the daily lives of those closest to her. She was still in ICU, still under 24 hour care. Sometimes it would be so busy in the ICU with other emergencies that hospital staff would leave Michelle's family or friends to watch over her, seeing as her condition was now the most stable of all ICU patients.

Michelle was running a bit of a temperature that was not responding to Tylenol. Her doctors suspected this was caused by damage to her inter-cranial temperature center, which was to be expected in a case such as this. A fan was directed on Michelle's body to keep her cool. Scott was still there on leave from his job in Nova Scotia. He gave Michelle a daily foot massage, which she seemed to enjoy.

Some of the nurses in the ICU were spectacular. The amount of tender care they gave Michelle went well beyond simply doing their job. These special people would moisten Michelle's mouth with mint swabs to keep her lips moist and fresh. Sometimes a nurse would brush Michelle's hair in a special way, or put lotion on her limbs with a gentle massage. Once in a while, a nurse would stop in Michelle's cubical and stay for a while, visiting with the family, talking to Michelle. Cori in particular appreciated the "little extras."

In the beginning of the second week of Michelle's stay in the hospital, she had two surgeries, the first being a tracheotomy in her throat so she could be ventilated, the second a gastrostomy, which would allow her to be tube fed directly into her stomach. Dr. Hayashi, the doctor who performed the tracheotomy, informed the family that there was a bit of a problem with Michelle's esophagus. There was a little tear in it because it was so small, but he assured them it would heal and not create a problem. It was wonderful for all to see her face completely free of medical tubes. The swelling in her lip began to recede. Her face went back to looking like Michelle. It was obvious to those around her that Michelle was aware of her surroundings. Her eyes were looking here and there. But there was no movement of her body. Nothing.

To everyone's delight, Michelle was completely removed from the ventilator and was breathing on her own. It was so exciting. Michelle could breathe!

• • •

Cori sat close to the side of the bed. Michelle's eyes were open. She seemed quiet, restful. Then Cori noticed a tear sliding down the side of Micelle's face. Cori dabbed the tear with her finger and held her sister's hand. They cried together. Cori felt unbelievably sad for Michelle. Yet, she also experienced a sense of delight that Michelle was able to display emotion.

"I think she (Michelle) was beginning to really understand the situation she was in. Perhaps she was relieved to be off the machine. But, it was the first time I really had seen her cry since it all began. I wasn't ever sure if that was because mentally she wasn't all there and couldn't feel emotion or if she was just being tough and denying the whole thing or what. So, when she cried it was like she was human and mentally I knew she was 'there', that she was thinking and processing it all. And bitter-sweet because I didn't want to see Michelle crying – that hurt me to see her upset."

• • •

Two good things happened then. Michelle was removed from antibiotics. And she was moved from the ICU to her new private room: room 605. The window of her room overlooked the parking lot. There were lots of trees and lots of sun. And there was even some view of the mountains. Scott and Tammi really missed Michelle's laugh, so one day they played a CD of music from South Park, one of Michelle's favorite shows. She started laughing, and they were thrilled. It was the first time in so many days that they finally heard something from her. Oh, but her face began to turn a bright red. In a panic, they immediately turned off the CD. It was too much stimulation too soon. Still laughing and, at the same time, feeling kind of bad, they snuck out of the room. After that, however, they would try different things to help Michelle respond. Because they now knew "she was there."

Dr. Carole Williams, a family physician who was called in, explained to the family and Michelle in simple terms what had happened to her. The condition was referred to as "locked in". Michelle's stroke had severely damaged her brain stem, the part of the brain that controls motor functions. However, Michelle's brain, the part that takes care of all thought processes, was mostly unharmed. Consequently, Michelle was unable to control her body, but maintained her full and complete faculties. Basically, her mind, her memories, her feelings, her hopes and dreams, were "locked in" to a body that could no longer respond to the commands of her brain. Dr. Williams knew that Michelle could respond 'yes' by raising her eyes upwards. The doctor asked Michelle if she had a headache. *Yes.* Then the doctor asked Michelle if she was scared. *Yes.* Dr. Williams gently responded, "I would be too."

Michelle was now developing an awful tape burn on her cheek. Nurses did their best to keep her as comfortable as possible by treating the burn with a salve.

Irene, an occupational therapist, looked in on Michelle and spoke to the family about the physical therapy they would be doing with her. One thing she suggested was getting Michelle a pair of high top sneakers for her feet for good support.

On Friday, May 28 Michelle celebrated her twenty fifth birthday. Family and friends did their best to make the most of it. Scott was catching a flight back to Nova Scotia that morning. He walked Michelle down to x-ray for an unscheduled CAT scan, said goodbye to her, and left with Gordon for the airport. Tammi gave Michelle a birthday card and was pleased when Michelle laughed. Kristy gave her a card also, which also inspired a laugh. A couple of hours later Scott returned, unable to catch a standby flight back home. He jokingly wrote in her diary, "Oh, darn." He was happy to spend a bit more time with Michelle. That day was a busy day for her, with all the company and lots of things happening with her care. Nurses gave her some Tylenol, then washed her hair. Michelle seemed to communicate with her eye movements that she was pleased. The physiotherapist also worked with Michelle's left side. And then, of course, Scott gave her his daily foot massage.

Michelle had been in the hospital for almost two weeks. It was time for Gordon and Joan to return home to Kamloops. They had responsibilities there that needed attention, and they now felt that Michelle was out of mortal danger. When they visited her that morning just before leaving to catch the ferry, Michelle seemed despondent. Was she upset because they were going? They didn't know. Michelle refused to respond to any of their questions. Later on, after her parents had left, Scott, being the character that he was, came up with a nose picking comment that got Michelle in a better mood. He was excited to see Michelle slightly moving her head. She even laughed at her new high top sneakers. The next day Scott had to say goodbye. It was a sad, sad moment. Then, as luck would have it, he once again could not catch a flight. He spent most of the day with Michelle. She was trying to move her arm. That was good.

• • •

The brain, being extremely complex, can cause all sorts of oddities in a person's behavior when it is damaged. Emotions of sudden outbursts of anger or deep and uncontrollable bouts of depression are quite common. When the brain has been altered in its delicate process of deciphering what is happening to the body it inhabits and the environment it is now experiencing, it often misfires and causes the person to do things out of character and, frighteningly for family, display odd and disturbing behavior.

Sandy Fulton explained it this way: "There were times when she (Michelle) could not NOT cry and that's a very normal reaction when a person has a brain injury. A lot of emotional stuff is in a certain part of your brain. But when the brain stem is hurt like it was, she doesn't have any control over her emotional thermostat. It's controlled by the hypothalamus actually. It's like when somebody has a stroke and they're crying all the time. I could be talking to you and have a stroke and all of a sudden I'd be crying and I'd have no idea why I'm crying. The hypothalamus is deep in the brain and it controls a whole bunch of things including emotions. So she'd be trying to express herself and then she'd be crying again and you knew she had no plan to cry. In the early days you can't control it. It would just be tears. And her little face would crumple. But you and I know that if something sad is happening we can go to a certain place and say 'okay, I don't need to react to this now'; so my thermostat of emotion went up and I said 'no no' you can go down and do something later. With a brain injury their thermostat is so out of whack, it's just like cry or laugh or something. You can't control it."

So, for Michelle, crying was very likely caused by her brain injury. She simply had no control over that particular emotion. Yes, she was probably frightened. Yes, she was probably terribly confused. But, when she cried, there was a good chance it was a medical problem that caused this emotion to come on spontaneously and for no particular reason.

Chapter 11

It was the beginning of the third week of Michelle's stay in VGH. Early in the morning she was given a chest x-ray. Her lungs were sounding unclear. Scott was staying at the girls' condo and took a phone call from a nurse at the hospital. She informed him that during the night Michelle's tracheotomy started to bleed and there were possible blood clots. They had taken her off of the blood thinning drug Heparin and were watching her very closely. Scott called the Britton's in Kamloops and informed Paul of the situation. All was okay. This information did not overly upset anyone back home. They were confident that Michelle was receiving the very best of care.

Occupational therapists helped Michelle sit up in bed. She had no control of her body and could not hold up her head. The therapists noted there were no adverse reactions and her positioning was good.

One of the hospital doctors, Dr. Dyson, stopped by to visit Michelle and had a talk with Scott who was visiting in her room at the time. They discussed the improvement in Michelle's ability to communicate; that her eyes were open most of the time now. Scott informed the doctor that Michelle was able to focus.

The following day Michelle had another chest x-ray. Valerie, a speech therapist reported that Michelle was responding well with eye movements and, on command, could follow an object with her eyes. That afternoon Scott dropped by for a visit and Michelle's parents arrived. They mentioned they were among the last five cars to make it onto the ferry. Lucky. But they had to patrol the hospital parking lot to find a space. They were happy when Michelle laughed a couple of times. Dr. Martin informed them that everything was going well with Michelle and that her CAT scan showed nothing abnormal. Dr. Waters came by and listened to Michelle's chest. Her lungs were sounding better and her chest x-ray was also clear.

Cori was visiting and asked Michelle if it was a good idea for her to go swimming. Michelle indicated *yes*. It was so difficult for Cori to leave her sister behind. Less than a month ago, Michelle and Cori were able to go together anywhere they wanted to. It was unbelievable that Cori now had to swallow her sadness and guilt and head off to do things her sister could not.

When Joan and Gordon arrived at the hospital the next day, they watched as student nurses performed daily care with Michelle. They washed her, performed mouth care, and re-positioned her. They cleaned her trachea and "restrung" it, and then suctioned out her lungs. Margaret, a physical therapist, came by to work with Michelle, but decided Michelle was too tired. She would work with her later. Michelle did not seem to be swallowing as much on this day, maybe because she was positioned on her side, which may have made it more difficult. Michelle was visited by Tammi and Scott. Dr. Martin was in and seemed pleased with how things were going. Martin Young, a social worker, had dropped by to meet the family.

When Michelle was placed on her right side, she seemed to want to turn her head to the left. Nobody really knew the significance of this. There was always so much guessing. Scott noticed that Michelle had a good grip when he held her hand, like she was squeezing. She held on so tight he could lift her arm. He also noticed some arm movement and some shoulder shrugging. What Scott didn't know was that "gripping" was a natural reflex and was not a voluntary movement on Michelle's part. Her shrugging, however, was a muscle movement she was totally doing herself.

When Cori and Kristy visited in the evening, they got Michelle laughing so hard she started coughing. The nurse reassured them this was good for her.

• • •

This was now Michelle's life. Oddly, she was not depressed. At this point Michelle did not fully realize the journey she was on. She was actually giddy, laughing, and all smiles. She became young minded, childlike. Her eyesight was terrible, but she could easily recognize family and individual caregivers by their voice and even by their gait. Improvements in her condition were miniscule, hardly noticeable. The daily care she received at the hospital became routine. Some mornings she would have a bath. Every day her trachea was cleaned. Physiotherapists would put Michelle through certain motions and sometimes help her sit up on the edge of her bed. This would totally exhaust her and leave her tired and less responsive. Visitors would sit quietly at those times and allow her to rest. Doctors would visit regularly, checking things like her oxygen level and her trachea. Tammi would often file Michelle's nails. And, of course, Scott would be there to provide moral support and a daily foot massage.

One of the very first things Michelle noticed when she became more alert and aware of her surroundings was how people would "talk over me" as though she actually wasn't there, or was not able to understand. She definitely did not like this. She needed to be recognized as more than just a patient. She was Michelle Britton. A human being. With thoughts and feelings!

It was almost three weeks into Michelle's stay at the hospital. Scott finally had to leave for Nova Scotia to return to work. He wrote a note for Michelle, "I will miss you big time." Michelle would not see him again for many months.

And so her daily life continued. The doctors had decided to cut back on some of the medications for Michelle's bowels and stomach and were to change her trachea in a few days. Cori visited her sister around the evening meal time and jokingly discussed how both of them had hairy legs. Sunday would be leg shaving day, for both of them.

It was noted the following day that half of Michelle's legs had been shaved. The other half would be done when she was turned over. Tammi painted Michelle's nails purple and someone had put her hair into a ponytail. Michelle was wide-eyed and laughing that morning. However, later in the day, she seemed sad and despondent. She was not responding to questions and put a sad expression on her face. Her dad started reading her a love novel, *The Notebook,* then played her some Beethoven. On that day she received a new airbed. A good airbed helps prevent both pressure points on the skin and very serious bed sores. Cori arrived in the late afternoon with Kristy. They visited and laughed for two hours straight. Cori thanked Michelle for a very positive evening.

It had come the time in Michelle's recovery to embark on serious goals. There was to be speech therapy, occupational therapy, and physiotherapy. Therapists asked family and friends to record all of Michelle's communicative responses such as smiles, eye blinks, or tears. Michelle would be trained to use these movements more consistently, thereby developing a useful communication system. Michelle was also coming along nicely with her body's handling of food. She had been on continuous feeding. Doctors decided it was time to give Michelle food with more fiber, and she would be fed every three to four hours in larger amounts. This would be closer to the regular feeding times most people were accustomed to.

Dr. Tina Webber, a resident doctor, asked Michelle if she wanted medication to help her be stronger in her moods. Michelle was told it would be a very low dosage. At this point Michelle declined the offer. So, it was decided they would wait and see how she managed.

• • •

Cori wrote this note to Michelle's speech therapist:

For Heather:

I hope you read this. I wish to speak with you personally and get some communication between us going. Michelle and I have always been best friends/close, almost twins. Sometimes, we don't even have to communicate; I know what she's thinking. Lately, I explored ideas with Shell. I know she can use her eyes more. Like for example, eyes rolled from left to right could mean "go away". Or a close of the eyes for a long time (a definite one) can mean change subject, etc. She also laughs to mean "yeah right!" (sarcasm) or "yes, of course it is!" depending on the context. Not just for jokes. She can also smile and purse (spelling?) her lips. We could work on these things. Also, I don't know what you use for "yes" but the "yes" I use for her works best. She is to open her eyes wide and tall so lots of white shows. I remind her that this (to me) is "yes" and then she uses it too if that's her answer. Also, "no" is not apparent to most of us. We think if there looks like a "no" answer, we should change the question around to get what we think "yes" would be the answer. Then, ask the "yes" question and she can confirm that that is what she wants. That is what works for me and I continue to tell mom and dad these thoughts. I am free next Wednesday, June 16th if we can meet! I would love to. Good luck with ETRAN.

Michelle's (only) sister, Cori

Chapter 12

For those who loved Michelle, it was now the small things in life that were noticed. Cori was aware of Michelle's ability to swallow. Some days Michelle would swallow quite often, other days not so much. Cori would hold Michelle's left hand and feel a tight grip, wondering if Michelle was doing this on her own. Cori saw that Michelle was wearing socks only, with no shoes. She made a point to bring Michelle more socks. Sometimes simply watching Michelle sleeping peacefully was enough to make Cori feel good.

Cori also loved to see a nice smile on Michelle's face, and her laughter was inspiring. She read Michelle the book *Imagine* which basically suggested that dreams can come true. Cori wasn't sure why this story caused Michelle to become silent. Maybe it was too strong a message for her at the time. That was one of the most stressful aspects of Cori's experience with her sister. Communicating with Michelle was hit-and-miss at best. Cori never knew for sure.

When she helped Michelle practice coughing and swallowing, Cori sensed that Michelle was happy to clear her own throat, but then it also looked like it hurt. She didn't know. Then Michelle sucked everything back with her next breath and had to be suctioned. Cori thought her sister was mad, annoyed, disappointed. She wasn't sure. But she did manage to make Michelle laugh when she suggested Michelle had permission to punch her in the stomach. Laughter was so good. But then a few hours later, Cori noticed her sister crying. Then Cori cried. The two of them played "cry-tag" for almost an hour. When they finally settled down emotionally, Cori read Michelle a couple of jokes. Michelle laughed, then fell asleep. Cori went home.

Cori wasn't sure, but she could swear Michelle moved the right side of her lip on her own, and also moved her head to the right. There were also movements that were worrisome. Michelle's arms and legs would tense up and Cori would massage them until everything relaxed. Also scary were the times when Michelle would laugh, then make a face like she had just violently coughed. These were all new things, unexpected things that could be somewhat startling.

Tammi also noticed the simple things. Holding Michelle's right hand she felt as if Michelle's hand was pushing quite strong. Michelle's "motor boat" lungs were now sounding crystal clear. Tammi massaged and creamed Michelle's hands and promised to change her nail color. It broke Tammi's heart to see her friend in this terrible condition. But she was determined to make the best of it. She would make sure Michelle always looked her best. She would help Michelle any way she could. She would help Michelle learn how to talk and walk and be the best she could be. No matter what, Tammi would always be there for her amazing friend.

Dr. Carole Williams made the decision to put Michelle on anti-depressants. It was unimaginable to the doctor that Michelle would be able to cope with the horror of her condition without some sort of calming medicine. She hoped an antidepressant would ease the distress.

It was a very changed life for everyone. Tammi would go to work; then go to the hospital. Cori would go to work; then go to the hospital. Joan and Gordon would stay at the girls' condo for days or weeks at a time, spending a good portion of their days with Michelle at the hospital. Scott would visit daily or, when he was back in Nova Scotia, call long distance to check on Michelle. Paul visited as often as he could manage.

Michelle herself would remain in her bed, hour after hour, day after day, adjusting to her new life. To Michelle, who was now becoming more aware of her surroundings, the days seemed very much the same: routine, monotonous, and endless. The small things she did on a daily basis were recorded by the professionals. Michelle *seemed* happy. Even though she tired after 20 minutes, she appeared to enjoy sitting in her big blue Broda wheelchair, a sort of Lazyboy chair on wheels. Her brightness and laughter were noted. Her smile had become more balanced on both sides of her mouth and her eyes were tracking better. She was placed in her bed at a higher angle of 45 degrees. She managed to occasionally cough up mucous on her own and avoid suction.

Therapists were definitely noticing improvements. When Michelle was placed in her chair she could even hold up her head a bit. One therapist, Heather, was working on getting Michelle to blink once for "yes" and blink twice for "no". It was questionable who was in control of Michelle's destiny. What therapists wanted, what Cori wanted, and what Michelle wanted, when it came to communication, went in different directions.

Family watched over Michelle very carefully. They observed therapy sessions, kept a close eye on any body movements, and were constantly on alert for anything that may cause her discomfort. For a few days it was observed that Michelle had a yellow coating on her tongue. Was it thrush? Nurses would keep an eye on it. It was noticed by Gordon that Michelle moved her head about one inch to the right. She also managed to hold up her head for about five minutes while in her chair. Fatigue was a big thing, however. Only a few minutes of therapy would drain her and she would spend the rest of the day resting and sleeping.

An exciting thing happened one evening. Cori was at home sick and could not visit Michelle, so a portable phone was brought into Michelle's room. Cori was able to talk to Michelle over the phone, and it was in everyone's mind that maybe Scott could now call her from Nova Scotia. They were thrilled at the prospect.

There were even better things happening the following day. Gordon was massaging Michelle's feet and asked if she could feel anything. Michelle replied with her eyes a definite "yes" to both feet. This gave her father much hope. Also, an alphabet sheet was presented to Michelle to test her knowledge of letters. Michelle identified "M' and "J" and "I Love U" on the board. She did this quickly and easily. It was obvious that she had retained her intelligence. No doubt! This was a fantastic breakthrough for future communication. Gordon and Joan were so hopeful, writing in Michelle's hospital journal, "Time will tell." When Cori visited later, she remarked on how Michelle's signals were so clear. "Awesome." Cori could also tell Michelle wanted to get rid of the trachea because she was trying very hard to cough up mucous on her own, even though it still appeared to hurt her.

• • •

Michelle was thinking much more clearly now, definitely coming out of her fog. Since her mind was so active, communicating with hospital staff and family was frustrating. Blinking her eyes for "yes" and "no" was tiring. And trying to get her point across to others was nearly impossible. The one thing she noticed from the very beginning, people "talking over her", was insulting. They often acted as if she wasn't there. This was especially true of some of the nurses.

The anti-depressants Michelle was on did not seem to make any difference to her mood. She was mostly bubbly and all smiles, and never really did feel she needed those kinds of drugs. She hated the suctioning of her lungs. It was very uncomfortable, yet it actually made her feel much better afterwards. When therapists sat her upright in a chair, she found it was very hard work and extremely tiring. It was not something she looked forward to in the beginning. Physiotherapy for her speech was disturbing. Her mouth and tongue just wouldn't work, no matter how hard she tried. She was very excited, however, when a tingling feeling began to return to her legs. This "verified her determination to improve."

And Michelle was very determined. When nurses would ask her to squeeze their hand, Michelle would try very hard to squeeze back, and when she was successful in doing this, she was very excited with her accomplishment. These were small, miniscule improvements. And, as Cori would write in the diary, "they were great."

Chapter 13

The family was diligent with writing in the daily diary in Michelle's room, keeping a record of the events of each day: who visited, and what their personal notes to Michelle were. Cori and her parents also made detailed observations on each improvement they noticed with Michelle. Cori began to rate each of Michelle's days from one to ten, "one" being a very low and difficult day and "ten" being an exceptionally good day where Michelle was energetic and alert and happy.

One day Gordon noted with an exclamation mark that when he touched Michelle's knees she laughed. This led him to believe she could now feel the sense of touch much higher in her legs. Michelle's parents were very encouraged by her ability to cough and swallow most of the time.

There were awkward, upsetting moments, however. They noticed that the position of Michelle's head seemed uncomfortable, kind of kinked up in the neck. They tried to rearrange her head, but felt bad when they couldn't achieve much. They couldn't seem to get it right. Cori visited later in the day and noticed that Michelle had moved her head to the right a few times. But when Cori asked her sister to move her head, Michelle didn't, or couldn't, do it. Cori chalked it up to Michelle being tired, although she was confident that Michelle was aware that she could move her own head. Cori rated this day a "six" day.

Many comments written in Michelle's diary were very positive. There was always excitement when Michelle showed any improvement in her communication skills. Michelle could now listen to Scott over the phone, and she would blink her eyes, open her eyes wide, and laugh and smile. Cori had asked Michelle to turn her head and look at her when she was finished with the phone call, and Michelle did it. Cori was so impressed with Michelle's new ability.

One of the nurses who sang along with a Reba CD was very surprised when Michelle lifted her head off the pillow and moved it back and forth to indicate "no" when asked if she need a Tylenol. Karen, one of the nurses, reported that Michelle moved her left toe on command. This news created a lot of excitement for Joan and Gordon.

Who would have thought such a small thing would mean so much?

The Brittons liked Karen, noting that Michelle was lucky to have Karen with her most of the day. The young nurse put a perfect French braid into Michelle's hair. That same day Tammi oiled Michelle's cuticles and painted her nails green. It was a very busy day. Physiotherapists had Michelle in her wheelchair and she was rolled down to the sunroom and back, a twenty minute excursion. Cori could see lots of movement in Michelle now. Michelle moved her head quite often from left to right and both of her legs were moving, especially her left one. Cori also noticed that Michelle was moving her jaw and mouth a lot. Did this mean Michelle would soon talk?

Dr. Waters dropped by to tell Michelle her tracheal tube would be changed for a different type of tube at the end of the week. He told her everything about the operation. Michelle cried. Even though she was pleased she was "finally moving in a positive direction," Michelle was also quite anxious about the surgery.

When the doctor left, she shed tears again.

Cori jotted down a few comments and feelings in her own personal diary: "This case is so different from all others. Apparently only 45 in the world. (Known cases. I'm sure there is a whole lot more just misdiagnosed). I'm not sure if any others have been at the brain stem, however...It is so frustrating for Mich. She understands, comprehends but can't respond like she wishes. It's frustrating for us, also. Watching and trying to help her but feeling helpless and incapable of making her get better. Hardest part is seeing her cry... Shell gets a new trach on Friday and it can be corked to see if she can talk. But, she can hardly move her neck and muscles there, so I'm not sure she could. No rush. She needs to heal. But, they have been sitting her up in a chair 15-25 minutes a day! And today, Mom and Dad wheeled her down to the sun room, past about 5-7 rooms, etc. I wish I had been there! And since, she's moving her left leg (a bit of her right as well). Her head also is moving a lot – like saying NO. Today was absolutely amazing. But then, she was super tired and cried. Just overwhelming, I suppose. She's also on Zoloft, an anti-depressant (one of Pfizer's). It's only a small bit/dosage a day but the thought of her needing them scares me, I guess... Everything is just very different right now. In such a short time."

• • •

Michelle's memory was completely intact, though it took some time for her brain to heal from its terrible trauma. What mainly interfered with her memory was the total concentration of her mind with her daily routine. In the hospital there was always something going on.

But as time passed, Michelle's medical schedule was less demanding. There was more time for her to think. And she would sometimes reminisce over some of the fun times.

Wallaper Lake brought her happy thoughts. The Brittons and two other neighborhood families would spend an early February weekend up at this lake every winter for about four years in a row. This meant that Michelle would spend the weekend with her best childhood friend, Adele. The three families would head out on a late Friday afternoon. They would all have dinner at a popular truck stop on the south side of Kamloops. Michelle would usually order a burger and fries.

Wallaper Lake Resort had about eight rustic cabins clustered off the side of the frozen over lake. Michelle and her neighbors would meet seven or eight other families there. This was a group of close friends who had met at church and church functions.

Michelle really liked those weekends. They were packed with so much fun and adventure that Michelle always felt it seemed much more than just two days.

On Saturday night the families rented the main lodge and had a potluck dinner. Michelle especially liked the Mexican Mess. This was a seven layer dip that included refried beans, guacamole, sour cream, and salsa, topped with grated cheddar cheese, tomatoes, and green onions. One of the dads would bring out his guitar and they would all have a sing along in front of the bonfire.

It was a very rustic experience. The cabins did not have running water or electricity. Each day they had to go down to a back room off the main lodge for water. There was also firewood to be hauled back to the cabin. Each cabin was one room with a wood stove, sink, table, and two double beds. They brushed their teeth using a cup of water and the sink. Hands and faces were washed in a big bowl of water. They could only see at night by using flashlights. And Michelle did not like having to use an outhouse. It was too cold and "not fun."

Most of those days were spent outside. The lake was completely frozen over and covered with about two feet of snow. They would cross country ski in the ski tracks already on the lake. They would skate and toboggan.

These sorts of memories were a comfort to Michelle, even though they evoked great sadness.

• • •

Nurses had sat Michelle in her Broda chair out in the hall for a while. This would totally exhaust her. Sitting upright was very tiring. So, most of her days were spent resting in bed. But her mind was becoming more and more active. She needed something to keep her mind busy.

Cori recognized that Michelle was bored. She asked Michelle if she would like to listen to story CDs and Michelle indicated she would like that. Cori would make sure her mom and dad and the nurses would know to turn on a CD for Michelle when she was left alone.

One particular thing Cori became aware of was that Michelle would open her eyes very wide when she desired to be left alone. Michelle was obviously indicating when she was too tired for a visitor.

Michelle did manage to sit up for about 25 minutes when her mom and dad took her on a tour of ward 'A' and ward 'B' of the hospital. Michelle seemed to enjoy the ride, watching as the nurse tried to entertain her with song and dance. Nurses Lisa and Diane were "awesome:" very energetic and helpful.

On June 25, forty one days into her hospital stay, Michelle had a new tracheal tube put in, and this one was 'corked.' This meant that Michelle could now breathe through her nose and mouth. This was great progress and Michelle was very happy with the change. Her throat felt more comfortable. Michelle didn't really understand why she "needed this thing in her neck." She thought she could do fine without it.

Dr. Dyson, the doctor who performed the tracheal surgery, told Michelle and her family that, if Michelle tolerated the corked tracheal tube, the tracheotomy would be completely removed and closed up in a week or so.

Cori recalls, "The new trach being corked meant another milestone passed. Baby steps I called them. Do this, then next comes this, and bit by bit…The corked trach meant that maybe now she could talk – up to this point, we didn't know because the trach was in and you can't really talk with that unless you temporarily close it and we had never tried that. So, would Michelle now talk? We weren't sure but it was a nice thought."

Lisa, the nurse, mentioned how happy Michelle seemed with her new tracheal tube. Lisa also noted that she had even heard Michelle's voice.

Cori was now hopeful that Michelle would soon be drinking from a cup. Cori was also trying her best to make sure Michelle's communications were understood by others. She wanted everyone to realize that Michelle could now turn her head from left to right in an obvious indication of "stop what you're doing right now" or "change the subject."

Cori knew that Michelle would thrive off good communication. It was Cori's devoted focus on her sister's various facial and head movements that inspired others to pay more attention to the young Michelle who was now locked in her body. Cori knew her sister would get better.

• • •

On June 22 Cori wrote in her diary: "Trach, G-tube, arterial dissection, suctioning, Zoloft, Coumadin, etc. All words I never thought I'd ever know about-EVER! It has been 5 weeks and Michelle is still in the hospital."

Cori also wrote about the personal changes in her life since Michelle's stroke: "Mom and Dad are basically living in our townhouse. Tammi has moved out early. I don't blame her. I need my space also but I can't afford it just yet. It's hard living with parents again. My life consists of working and hospital with a bit of swimming and going to the gym. Fun? Not so much. I'm usually too tired to go out or plan things with 'friends.' What are friends, by the way? It all comes down to family, basically. My friends are all living in different parts of the world. The ones here in Victoria are not helping too much. They don't know what to do."

Another note in Cori's diary eluded to her confusion with her new daily life: "Sometimes, when I have the feeling that I just wish to be alone, and I get to be alone, I don't like it. I feel lonely! Isn't that ridiculous? Am I mixed up, to want company and not want company at the same time? How many others feel this way, I wonder? I think I'm just going to sit here awhile and watch the lights and the ocean."

Chapter 14

Dr. Carole Williams had a meeting with the family, including Michelle. The doctor discussed plans for Michelle's future with B.C. Rehab. It was a frank discussion and Michelle was teary, obviously upset with her grim life ahead: days and weeks and months of exhausting physiotherapy.

But later on that day Michelle began experimenting with her vocal chords. She would hear a noise from her voice and would do it over and over. She laughed at her new ability. Cori thought this different challenge for Michelle was motivating. Michelle was fighting to get better.

The nurses were so good to Michelle. They bathed her and would nicely braid her hair; they would put cream on her entire body and put lip gloss on her lips. If Michelle's throat was sore they would give her Tylenol. They would do their best to keep Michelle happy and upbeat. The nurses would also sometimes write in her diary, commenting on the events of the day and how often she would chuckle and laugh.

There were certain personal tasks the nurses did with Michelle, taking care of the bowel, cleaning all areas of her body. This was a time when Cori was content to let others take over. "The nurses always made us leave when private things were being done. For the most part, I was totally fine with that – for Michelle's dignity mostly, but also I didn't wish to see it all. I didn't mind caring for her but not the private things."

Cori had a great time with Michelle one evening when they laughed non-stop for about two hours. A friend was giving Michelle a sob-story when Michelle seemed to let out an "aw" with her voice. Cori also thought Michelle tried to say "I" once, and was certain that Michelle was "definitely experimenting with her voice when not tired." Cori was also helping her sister work on her wink. Cori guessed the wink could mean "thank you." But, again, she wasn't sure.

Michelle was gaining strength and stamina. She was now sitting up in her chair for up to 45 minutes. And she loved getting out of her room, even though it was a major exercise in patience for her to get comfortable in her chair. It was completely draining. But Michelle knew it was necessary for her to forge ahead. Her speech therapist, Heather, would sit in the sun room with Michelle and they would practice exercising her facial movements. It was a huge task for Michelle to move her tongue over her bottom teeth.

The importance of the tongue in the human body is not something that would concern the average 25 year old adult. Few pay attention to the fact that the tongue is needed to chew food, swallow, or sing. And without the tongue it is impossible to taste or talk. The tongue is an assortment of muscles. The flexible front part of the tongue works with the teeth in creating words. This part of the tongue also helps move the food around in the mouth while chewing. Muscles in the back of the tongue help to make certain sounds like "k" or "q". These back muscles are also very important for swallowing. They help push food down the esophagus.

In Michelle's new life she became highly aware of the intricacies of the body's various muscles. Suddenly, what before came naturally and almost unnoticed, was now an almost impossible challenge. The frustration was indescribable. But, what could she do? She couldn't yell or scream or swear. She couldn't pound her fist or stomp her feet or punch a pillow. She could only lay there, motionless, and cry.

Another thing Michelle had to deal with was pain. Sometimes she would wince when moved, and then she would cry. Nurses suspected Michelle's crying was a sign that she was very uncomfortable. Dr. Williams prescribed Tylenol to be administered every four hours, which seemed to help Michelle with being moved and positioned.

On July 1st, Canada Day, it was reported that Michelle was brought some clothes to wear in place of her blue hospital gown. She now had a choice of green boxer shorts, white boxer shorts, her favorite sweat shirt, and a new purple T-shirt. Michelle often practiced moving her mouth and could now open it really wide and almost stick her tongue out. She also "moved her head on command and shrugged her left shoulder on command." Cori wrote in the diary: "Whooppee-progress!"

Understanding Michelle, especially for Cori, was getting a bit easier. One evening while Cori was visiting, Michelle was distraught, not responding, but definitely listening. Finally she started crying. Cori tried joking with her about PMS, however, Michelle made it clear to Cori she was in physical pain in the head. After being given Tylenol, Michelle's demeanor improved and she was ready to listen to a CD. She was also wondering if she someday be allowed to watch some TV.

It was strange the way certain moments with Michelle were so similar to those with a newborn. When Gordon sat with his daughter and held her hand, he was thrilled when she squeezed tight. He would often read to her, as a father would read a nighttime story to his little girl. Gordon would always be encouraged with any small improvement in Michelle's motor skills. But, being a realistic person, he accepted the fact that Michelle would most likely be very limited. He would sometimes be angry with God, wondering how He could allow such a terrible thing to happen to his innocent child. Was this really the loving God he had come to know through his church? It was so unfair. So cruel.

Scott would call on the phone once in a while. Michelle's face would brighten when she listened to his voice. He would talk to her for fifteen minutes or so and would tell Michelle all that was happening in his life in Nova Scotia. Cori was amazed with Michelle's facial expressions when listening to Scott. Cori had no idea what he was saying, only that it was "a million things" because Michelle was laughing, smiling and even opening her eyes really wide as if to say "Wow, really, oh my gosh!"

It was time, according to Lisa, a registered nurse, for Michelle to have moderate stimulation with TV. Michelle could also watch videos on the VCR. She was very happy with this.

Michelle was experiencing a few health problems due to her physical condition. Because she was not eating or drinking, her tongue was prone to yeast infection. The nurses painted her tongue with something that combated this. Michelle was also given Mycostatin for a bladder infection. And Dr. Williams was treating her for headaches.

Gordon and Joan took Michelle in her Broda chair down the corridor to the windows beyond the patient elevators. But Michelle could not stand the brightness of the sunlight. Joan made a note to bring Michelle a hat and sunglasses.

When Cori came into the hospital for her evening visit she was so sad for her sister. Poor Michelle was in her room with the curtains closed, no music, and no visitors. Cori thought "it seems so awful!"

Cori strongly felt a lack of control over Michelle's situation. She wondered if Michelle was having her shoes put on as regularly as before. It seemed a small thing. But Cori wanted her sister to have constant care and attention.

Watching TV with Michelle had to be very controlled. Michelle could only handle about ten minutes of this type of stimulation. For the present, there could be no sound or subtitles. Subtitles were just "too quick for Shell." Cori swabbed Michelle's mouth with a mint/water swab and helped Michelle practice swallowing, opening her mouth and sticking out her tongue. Another thing Cori would do is spend time with her sister looking at photos and reading Scott's emails.

When it came to over-stimulation with Michelle, Cori found it hard to describe. "Michelle would start to disengage with my conversation. Her face was always pretty animated and it usually isn't hard to know what she was thinking. But when there were so many things around her, all the people in the hallways, the sounds, the actions, etc., sometimes her eyes would start to gloss over, her face would be less respondent, and she would seem very tired. I don't know how to describe it but I knew that she was getting too much stimulation, like her brain was working overtime."

• • •

It was day fifty two of Michelle's stay in the hospital when it was decided that she could now venture outdoors. It was a beautiful sunny day. Tammi wheeled her out into the sunshine. Michelle was amazed with the freshness of the air, the pleasant smell of the trees. It was wonderful. The two of them just relaxed and watched the bunnies hopping around the grounds. It was a time when Michelle realized how people lived their lives way too fast and did not take the time to slow down and enjoy the simple things. She heard a helicopter and looked towards the sky. She laughed and remembered.

• • •

It was Scott who had introduced Michelle to planes and flying and she was instantly hooked. When he took her flying over Vancouver Island, she was amazed at how many wonderful sights she could see in such a short period of time. They flew many times together.

Michelle decided she wanted to learn how to fly and took night courses once a week. She would fly with an instructor on the weekends. It was a challenge sometimes for her to go to the flying class after a full day of university. But she loved planes and it was exhilarating to fly. Scary and exciting.

She recalled one flight with Scott and another friend. They were flying over Vancouver Island and Scott decided to stall the plane. This was an exercise of purposely stalling and restarting in the air. Michelle had done this before with Scott, so wasn't alarmed. It was above Mount Arrowsmith where Scott performed the exercise, but this time the plane wouldn't start. They were losing altitude fast, yet somehow Michelle didn't really panic and believed Scott would get it started. The mountainside grew closer and closer, then she suddenly felt the welcomed vibration of the plane's engine.

Later on Michelle did two solo flights, just her and the plane. She was nervous, but she knew she could do it. A thorough walk around the plane proved to her that the plane was ready to go. She listened to the radio and, following radio instruction, taxied and took off. That was the easy part. She did a circuit above the airport and then landed. It was not a pretty landing. She equated it to big grasshopper leaps down the runway.

Her second solo was smooth and uneventful. She felt powerful up there in the sky. Very confident. It was "a neat feeling" for Michelle to know she was controlling the plane.

And she thought, "It's a good thing I wasn't flying when I had the stroke."

• • •

In July, Dr. F. Killian wrote a consultation report:

Thank you for asking me to see Ms. Britton in consultation, whom I saw today, July 19, 1999.

She is a young woman of 25 years of age who on May 17, 1999, was found in the UVic parking lot. She had pre-existing history of headaches of 4-5 days duration and subsequently vomited. She was unconscious on arrival at the Emergency Room. An LP was described as normal and the consideration was that she had a vascular lesion and subsequently that it was likely a vertebral artery dissection.

An MRI was reported as showing lesions in the pons, right cerebellum and both thalamic areas. She required traching and was in the Intensive Care Unit initially.

At this time, she is on medication including Zololf 15 mg a day Serax, Tylenol extra strength, Coumadin.

At this time she is not on long term ventilation. She requires a feeding tube.

She is alert, responds to stimuli including, touch and the voice.

She appears to communicate with her eyes with yes and no but when she fatigues, this becomes inconsistent.

She remains totally dependent, shows poor head control and general flaccidity of the body. She has a poor cough but is starting to clear some secretions and does require regular suctioning.

She is breathing independently and moving her eyes.

She is placed in a Broda chair for seating and requires the use of a lift to transfer.

The bowel and bladder are functioning and are totally dependent at this time.

The goal of intervention is to continue to maintain good skin care with regular turning and appropriate positioning both in seating and in bed so that general hygienic care is easily maintained.

To continue on a bowel and bladder program. Therapy is to stimulate swallowing and head control at this time continuing with passive range of movement and safe transfers. At this time, the main function is maintenance and Michelle requires placement in appropriate setting at this time. She is only 2 months post insult, there is some potential for improvement in swallowing and head control, which may permit some use of environmental controls in the long term but the insult may have been significant that there is no evidence of change from flaccidity even in 8 weeks, which would be a poor prognostic indicator for future long term gains, with regards to her function.

Chapter 15

When Michelle was nineteen years old she lived at the international youth hostel in Kamloops. She worked a few shifts a week there in turn for free accommodation. She had her own personal area at the back right side of one of the hostel rooms. She had the use of one bunk bed and a set of shelves. The extra bunk was handy for storing her stuff. There was a communal bathroom downstairs and upstairs a kitchen. The hostel was close enough to the college that Michelle could walk to school.

There were four young adults living in this hostel, Michelle and three guys. Kevin and Mark worked in night security and Mick did odd jobs. Michelle's main job was to work the front desk doing reception. She would occasionally clean bathrooms or the kitchen or the sleeping rooms.

The building was an old historical courthouse. Beside the kitchen was a large open room with a wooden judge's bench and a jury box. Off this room was a small TV room, where one wall was fully lined with books. Michelle thought it was a majestic, "really neat" building with interesting back stairways and nooks and crannies.

It was a crazy time. Michelle met many people and made connections with travelers from all over the world. On her past trip to Fiji she had spent eight days with an English fellow. He came to see her at the hostel in Kamloops and she was able to show him around a bit.

Michelle loved to be around men. Mark, tall and dark-blond and lean, was into guitar and tried to teach Michelle how to play. For some reason, though, Michelle never could successfully tackle the instrument. Maybe her being left handed still posed too much of a challenge. She and Mark hung around together for about two months, mostly at the hostel. They didn't really go out much. Michelle liked his kindness and appreciated his need to protect her from the advances of other guys who were constantly surrounding her. He was quite jealous.

Adam, with his fake blond hair, was a shorter guy, almost stocky. He was from the States, and was traveling with Phillip. He was a nice looking young man, but Michelle was not really attracted to him. She thought it was smart of him when he purchased a balaclava for the cold winter ski slopes in Sunpeaks, the nearby skiing area. A lot of skiers stayed at the hostel.

Phillip, a tall dark haired guy, was from New Zealand. She didn't actually get to know him well, even when she later stayed with him and his parents in New Zealand. She remembered him as being solid, even-tempered, and could actually be quite funny. There was never anything romantic between them. He did teach her how to make falafels and chamomile tea.

Then there was Julian. He was traveling with a group of excursion students and stayed at the hostel for a while. Later on he rented a basement suite up the street from the hostel. Michelle joined Julian and a couple other guys at the Kamloops Climbing Gym where he taught her how to rock climb. Michelle and Julian had quite a few little adventures. One time they were at the college pub, meeting some of his nurse friends. He took Michelle home later on his bicycle. Michelle sat on the seat while Julian stood on the pedals steering the bike. Off they went down Columbia Street and First Street, two very steep hills. It was a wild ride, with no helmets to protect them. They were young and carefree.

Glen was a young man Michelle met at college through friends. He was average height and rode a bike for sport, so had a very good build. The interesting thing about Glen was he wrote a sex column for the college paper. Sex was very important to him, and he often practiced with Michelle - to her benefit. Michelle thought he was fun. She went to a couple of parties with him. There was one party where Michelle had smoked a lot of pot from a bong Glen had made. They drove back to the hostel and Glen, feeling so sick, slept on the couch by the bathroom downstairs. At these times, Michelle felt relaxed, and relieved from the pressures of school.

This seemed to be the way with Michelle and her friends, experimenting with life, careless and carefree; learning from each other through times of outdoor exploring, drinking and dancing at the bars, parties and pot, and a few sexual flings. Every day was so much adventure. So much fun. Michelle was doing it all.

• • •

Dr. Waters came by Michelle's room and commented on how beautiful she looked that morning. He then told her that her trachea tube would be removed the next day.

Michelle had a usual day, spending a half hour in her chair outdoors. The weather was not that nice, but she seemed to enjoy the fresh wind. Margaret was working with Michelle's legs and Michelle was pushing her left leg quite well. Cori commented that soon her sister would be walking. "Yeah."

In the early evening Cori was with Michelle and noticed that the earphones on the television were working. That was good news. Cori swabbed Michelle's mouth with lots of water and hoped she would be drinking out of a cup soon. Her visit that day ended with Michelle crying, using her only means of communication that would let people know she was in pain and needed Tylenol.

The following morning Michelle's trachea tube was removed. The hole in her throat was left to heal on its own, without any stitches. It was expected to completely close itself within 24 hours.

It was amazing how such a simple event in Michelle's care led to everyone feeling happy and optimistic. Her friends and family could suddenly envision a bright future for Michelle. They could see her bike riding again. They would listen to the funny sounds she made with her voice and could imagine her talking again.

All in all, it was a good experience for everyone, especially Michelle, who "laughed up a storm" while watching episodes of "Frasier" and "Friends." It was a high stimulation day for Michelle and she handled it well.

But the next day Michelle had a bit of a setback. She was not able to cough up mucus from her lungs because her throat was still sensitive, and an x-ray showed she had a bit of pneumonia. The physiotherapy people worked very hard on her chest to loosen things up, so Michelle was very tired, too weary to take her daily excursion in her chair. She was put on oxygen because her oxygen level was too low.

Daily suctioning was an important part of Michelle's care. Cori described it this way: "Yes, I watched as they suctioned, at first to make sure she was still good afterwards and then later I watched so that I could possibly do it for her when others (nurses) weren't available. I hated hearing her breathe with a raspy voice, knowing she needed suctioning, but I couldn't do it and we had to wait for someone. I remember us family soon learned how to do it because we knew she needed it often. It was gross to do it at first, then I felt good about doing it because it was so much clearer after. After suction, I always imagined her feeling so much better because it had been done. I know though, that she didn't like it. I can't imagine what it felt like having a little vacuum cleaning out your airways. The sound…I remember going to the dentist within that first year and having my mouth suctioned after the cleaning and hating it because it reminded me of Michelle's suctioning. The sound is exactly the same as at the dentist's."

Cori knew Michelle was not happy. She guessed Michelle had had a scary and painful day. She was receiving steam to loosen stuff up. Cori recorded that her sister had a "3" day.

A few days later physiotherapists noticed Michelle, while sitting in her chair, would lose her head position when she coughed. The therapists provided Michelle with an elastic strap to support her head back into the head support. They also provided Michelle with a wedge on her foot rest to help stretch her heal chords.

A psychiatrist from the G. F. Strong rehabilitation hospital briefly assessed Michelle and agreed to refer her to G. F. Strong, but likely in 6 months.

A few days later Michelle was definitely better. She indicated that her throat was less sore. Her mouth was loose and flexible. Her head could be moved to the left much further. She was coughing, swallowing and spitting very well. Michelle even let out a strong cough and spit right on Cori's face about a foot away. Of course, this did not upset Cori, but, rather, pleased her very much. And when Michelle laughed for about 10 minutes, bringing herself to happy tears, Cori was totally freaked out with the excitement. Things were getting better. Michelle was now making lots of sound with her voice. She was doing everything better.

Michelle's throat healed within 3 or 4 days and the bandage was removed. Her catheter was removed, so she no longer had a "pee-bag." This meant, however that she now wore a "big bed pan, diaper thing." And she hated it. She did not like being wet.

• • •

Every day, energy permitting, Michelle sat in her chair in the hallway for at least an hour or so. She didn't really like just sitting there, but preferred it to being tucked away in her room. She was able to see and watch the nurses do their work. Unfortunately, she could hear them too. And she sometimes didn't care to hear other people's conversations. Most of the time nurses were talking to each other about their patients, and Michelle would think it was none of her business to listen in. One day when she was sitting there in the hall she really questioned if that was going to be her life. "Nothing but hospital life."

Cori was leaving for a five day event, the Merritt Mountain Music Festival. Of course, Michelle was unhappy that she herself couldn't go. Even though country music wasn't her favorite, she would have enjoyed the vibe of the entertainment. It was a sad and frustrating time for Michelle.

It disturbed Joan and Gordon when their daughter was in pain. It seemed that Michelle was having trouble with the position of her neck. One time when Michelle had her head turned to the right to watch TV, she coughed and her head jerked to the left. This made her cry. Her parents did their best to position her more comfortably, which seemed to help Michelle settle down.

Joan and Gordon spoke with Katherine Cox, the Placement Liason. They signed papers to begin the process of moving Michelle to Extended Care. The target was to have her moved to Gorge Road Hospital where she would stay until she qualified for rehabilitation at G.F. Strong.

Michelle's parents wheeled her out to the sunroom and talked to her about moving. Even though Michelle was not happy with the topic, Joan and Gordon knew it had to be discussed. Michelle was very nervous, and dreaded moving to another facility, just another hospital; getting used to new routines and new caregivers. Gorge Road did not sound like the ideal place to go.

• • •

Tammi tried to visit Michelle every day. It was grueling, going to work, driving to the hospital, going to work, driving to the hospital. When Michelle's parents came from Kamloops, they stayed at the townhouse with Tammi and Cori. It was hard for Tammi to believe that an active person like Michelle, who was getting her pilot's license, who white water rafted, who rock climbed, would not be able to do that anymore. "It was just like…it was hard."

Although Tammi had heard about Scott, she had not met him until his first visit with Michelle at the hospital. Tammi and Scott wound up spending a lot of time together and she got to know him. She thought "he's great…he's a great human being." She could see that Scott and Michelle had exact personalities.

Tammi figured the relationship between Scott and Michelle could have been a very good one. The timing just wasn't right. When Scott and Michelle were dating, Scott was definitely not ready to get married. Tammi thought Michelle's visit with him down in Nova Scotia was "kind of a closure thing" for Michelle, a chance for her to "see his environment." Michelle had told Tammi that she and Scott had a really good time together. Tammi thought that was great and what both Michelle and Scott needed. Tammi looked at it from the perspective, "People move on and figure stuff out."

When Tammi visited Michelle she at first did not know how to respond to the way her friend seemed so much "not herself," even though Tammi "didn't think anything differently," that Michelle was still Michelle. Tammi knew "it was going to be a work in progress." But she didn't realize how much damage had been done to Michelle. All Tammi could do was think positively and that "we were going to have to work at it."

From the beginning of the whole ordeal, Tammi definitely did not think Michelle would die. She knew it was going to be a slow recovery process "because you never know about this kind of stuff, right. It's something new for everybody."

Tammi thought back to before Michelle's stroke: "I didn't even know it was a stroke that was happening. There was a migraine headache that she had for 5 days prior and we all told her…I went out to dinner with her the night before it happened and she said, 'my neck's been sore,' and I said, 'it's probably stress because you have exams coming up and you have to get your degree and I know what you're like because you're trying to make sure you get this done.' I said, 'Why don't you go to the doctor tomorrow morning and see if they can look at you and check it out.' Well, she dropped Cori off at work and that was it, right in the parking lot…so, they couldn't have found it because of how small it was and the location. It was a fluke. I can't even explain it. The way they explained it to me is that she could have been doing something, overhead painting, and jerked her head the wrong way, or somebody was roughhousing with her, tickling her…they just don't know."

Chapter 16

On the top of the page of July 19 in Michelle's diary is written, "9 weeks in hospital. Start of 10th."

Joan and Gordon had an appointment at the Gorge Rd. Extended Care Unit. Social worker, Jenny Aiken, took them on a tour of the place. It was about a forty minute meeting where they discovered there was a six month to one year waiting list. Upon return to Victoria General Hospital, they discussed this with social worker, Sandy Fulton. Sandy insisted there was nowhere else for Michelle, that she would have to stay at VGH.

Once again, while visiting their daughter, Michelle's parents noticed she seemed uncomfortable and in pain. Michelle was crying and moaning. They repositioned her. That was all they could do.

That same day Cori returned from the music festival. Michelle had a big smile on her face when she saw her sister, and seemed to listen in good spirits as Cori told her all about the entertainment. When it came to communication, Cori continued to make Michelle blink, even though Michelle seemed to want to open her eyes wide for "yes." Was Michelle exercising a need for independence?

Communicating with Michelle was still very uncertain. When Michelle indicated she had a stomach ache and a headache, hospital staff thought she could possibly be hungry. When she was fed, she seemed better. It was definitely a guessing game.

Cori and three others visited Michelle that evening and were laughing and joking. In Cori's mind, Michelle was "getting all the jokes." And, when Michelle wanted to watch TV, she would stare at it, suggesting someone turn it on for her. Cori remarked, "Holy communication!! It was perfect. She was happy."

One day Cori arrived at the hospital with Javier, a young Mexican man she was teaching in her "English as Second Language" class in a little school located in downtown Victoria. Cori could tell Michelle enjoyed seeing a handsome man and hearing a different accent. Javier would write in Michelle's diary quite often, in Spanish. He became an important person in Cori's life. Michelle really liked him. The relationship between Javier and Cori would last over two years. Michelle was sad when it eventually ended.

On another visit, through a special personal communication between them, Cori understood that Michelle's problem with pain was a stiff neck. Cori was relieved it was not a serious neurological problem. She helped Michelle practice her "p" and "f" sounds, and they worked on spitting, swallowing and coughing.

Cori noted with excitement, "We understand each other SO well!"

Another thing that both Tammi and Cori were working on was Michelle's ability to wink her left eye. Tammi thought this eye movement could be used to improve communication, using it as a way of saying something…maybe. "I don't know."

It was frustrating that there were no simple ways of finding out exactly what Michelle needed. Sometimes Michelle had a headache because she was thirsty and was dehydrated. Cori wanted to be sure her sister was receiving regular physiotherapy, but without directly asking Michelle, she could never be sure. She did manage one day to understand from Michelle that her sister had not received the daily moving of her legs or arms. And this was unacceptable to Cori. Michelle could not improve without regular therapy every single day. Cori tried so hard. How could she be there every single moment? She would have to have a very serious talk with Michelle's caregivers.

• • •

An acquaintance of both Cori and Michelle dropped in for a visit. Cori could sense that this person was out of sorts with seeing Michelle this way and didn't quite know what to do. Cori even suspected that Michelle was also aware of this uncomfortable feeling. The uneasy visitor left without staying very long. Cori noted, "It's too bad." Some people could deal with a person who was severely neurologically impaired, some just could not.

A few more small improvements happened over the next few days. Michelle could sit up in her chair for up to two hours now. And she could hold up her head by herself for 20 minutes. Michelle's leg would sometimes extend automatically and family encouraged her to relax it downwards. And she did it!

One time, when Cori was playing a Neville Brothers tape, Michelle became very upset, sobbing hard. Through a series of very specific questions, Cori found out that the song reminded Michelle of a friend from high school, Barb, who had died in a car crash. "Barb was great," Michelle recalled. "She wasn't well liked because she could be pushy and annoying but we were good friends. Barb's mother had her very young and her stepbrother was two. She lived near me in the next subdivision so I could easily walk over, which I often did. I didn't know her very long, mainly grade ten. Barb was my party buddy. We went to a few house parties and liked boys. I remember she made me a birthday cake. She was a year older so her car accident was after her Graduation." Michelle remembered how absolutely devastated she was when she received the phone call and was told her friend had died. Michelle's mom had been sitting in the living room and Michelle could barely move herself away from the phone to tell her mom about Barb's sudden death. Now, years later, it seemed a positive thing that Michelle maintained a good degree of emotions, yet it was sad that she had to suffer the internal pain.

Michelle was moved again, this time to the room next to the sunroom. It was a bigger space. Gordon, Joan, Cori and Tammi all helped to organize Michelle's things. Michelle was giving input as to where she would like things, and she seemed happy with her new environment.

Michelle was now turning her head both left and right. This was exciting progress for the nurses. Michelle was receiving less medication, Extra-Strength Tylenol every 6 hours for pain, a minimum dose of Zoloft balancing her moods, and, of course, Coumadin, a necessary blood thinner. "Not bad!"

• • •

Michelle liked her physiotherapists, Margaret and Trigg. They were lots of fun. Trigg, a guy who Michelle guessed was in his forties was the one who most liked to have fun. He told Michelle jokes or a story. Sometimes he would play music and dance, before Margaret came in. Margaret was a firm but sweet lady. She and Trigg were like an old married couple, even though they weren't married. It was with these two therapists that Michelle began serious therapy. They were there from the very start of Michelle's battle to hold up her own head. Margaret would remove the headrest and would hold Michelle's head with her hands. Michelle recalled waiting some time before she received a chair to sit in. After lying in bed so long, it was such a chore for her just to sit up.

• • •

It would have been interesting for Trigg and Margaret to have heard stories of Michelle's extensive travels to places all over the world. Michelle had written a diary of her first overseas vacation, a student exchange program, to France:

"Well we've already flown from Vancouver to Toronto and I'm on the way to Paris from Toronto. The first ride went quickly… Once in Paris we met our tour guide, Edith, and our bus driver Jean-Francois. We hopped on the bus and went to a Cathedral and champagne cellar in Reims…We arrived at our hotel in Selestat…I only slept for half an hour on the plane and I was tired but I couldn't sleep.

"The scenery is unbelievably different. On one side it will be totally flat and the other side will be mountainous. The towns are small with narrow crooked little streets and many cemeteries in the towns. The houses and buildings are very old and dirty. To sum it up: It's like Quebec – narrow streets; Vancouver – weather; Victoria – some of the trees; P.E.I. – rolling hills.

"Today we went to see the Haut-Koenigsbourg Castle way up on a hill. It was so neat! Then we went to Strasbourg near the German border. Once there we had lunch at a "flunch" (fast lunch or cafeteria) then started a walking tour. We went to see a cathedral and climbed 328 stairs up to the top of it and looked out. The view was excellent. On the left side you could see Germany! Then after going to the Post Office we had an hour and a half to roam the streets and go shopping. Cori, Shauna, Adele and I set off on a little tour. Then everybody took a scenic route back to our bus and came back to the hotel in Selestat for dinner…It was rainy today."

After a few days of traveling to smaller towns in France, young Michelle and her tour group ventured into Paris.

"It was windy and cloudy…headed for Paris…arrived in Paris and WOW was it incredible; people were everywhere!...We got out at Notre Dame and walked to a restaurant to eat…headed for a bank and souvenir shop…The guys here all turn to stare! It's fantastic!!...After that we went to the best ice cream shop in the world!... on to Notre Dame. It was so crowded! But it was beautiful…took a bus tour and stopped at a duty free shop where I bought some lipstick…Then it was on to meet the families."

The youths in Michelle's entourage were then to each stay for a few days with a French family. Michelle wrote about this experience along with meeting Isabelle, a French girl around her same age.

"Well, I'm with a girl whose father is a retired train engineer and her mother is an accountant. She has a sister who's 35 and married and has 3 kids! Isabelle seems to like horses. She goes riding every Friday and has many pictures of them! The house is extremely small but nice. I must admit I'm a little nervous and homesick (at least I wish I was with someone from the group!) For dinner we had chicken then we watched some T.V. I gave them gifts then we went to bed! They're nice people.

"It was rainy…My first full day with my family!...Isabelle and I then went into town…Isabelle and I went to visit her friend…We all walked through the park and saw the view of Paris…We went to the mall. It was 3 floors!...had fish, potatoes, bread, salad and yogurt for dinner. The fish was really good!"

Some of Michelle's writings showed her immaturity, for she was only about 15 or 16 years of age at the time of this vacation. She was most definitely keen on the opposite sex.

"Today I'm going to school with Isabelle from 10-11…really sunny out today!...The guys at her school are gorgeous but most of them smoke…Went with her to her gymnastics…Her gymnastics coach and P.E. teacher is very young and good looking!...Oh, by the way, I saw Lisa this morning. What a snob! She was sort of nice but I guess its just the way she is!...Isabelle and I went to the pool because she had to get a shirt from her friend. Well, her friend was gorgeous!! (tanned, dark hair) and there was another guy teaching at the pool, too! He had sandy blonde hair and a gorgeous tan!"

It was interesting how Michelle viewed the incredible sights of Paris, through the eyes of a young, blossoming adult.

"WOW! Today was exhausting!...we went to the bank then to the Louvre…Once inside we wandered around sort of lost and it was really a dumb system they had, but we saw the Mona Lisa and Michelangelo's sculptures and then left fairly quickly…started walking toward the Arc de Triumph. On the way there we ran into 2 guys from Montreal!...went under the Arc de Triumph. What a riot! We saw a lady with floral print nylons (how gross!) and then a guy with a real patch of RED hair. It all looked so funny!...headed for the Eiffel Tower…went up. WOW! What a view! You could see everywhere!"

Michelle's love of global travel throughout her late teens and early twenties most likely began with this very first vacation abroad. Her final comment in the diary hints of her newly acquired addiction. She writes, "I think I'll miss Paris!"

Chapter 17

Michelle was disgusted with her diaper. She would be left for hours with the discomfort and wetness. She would hold her bladder much longer than she should in order to avoid this embarrassment. The only way she could let people know she wanted to be "cleaned up" was to cry. Crying was her main way of communicating her needs. But it would sometimes seem to take forever for her caregivers to figure it out. Cori was a great help. She would "after a bit" learn what Michelle wanted and, before long, the problem would be solved and the sisters would spend valuable time together, with lots of laughing.

Tammi was such a wonderful friend to Michelle. She visited as often as she possibly could and fussed over Michelle's hair, or did her nails in all sorts of vibrant colors. Tammi and Michelle had always gotten along so well. Tammi could say she and Michelle had "never had an argument." Once in a while, especially during their Banff experiences, Tammi would really have choice words for some of Michelle's endless variety of boyfriends and would probably say "Like, why are you doing that, that's ridiculous." She worried that the guys were using Michelle. Tammi realized that her instinct to protect Michelle was just part of her own personality, an unexplainable need to help her close friend. She didn't want Michelle to do something that was going to hurt her in the end.

Joan recalled medical staff telling her, from the very beginning of Michelle's ordeal, that the family must try to focus on looking after themselves: take a break, go for a walk. Michelle had many visitors, so Joan found herself often in the waiting area where she sort of "took over" the room, sometimes reading, sometimes working on the ongoing jigsaw puzzle. Joan thought this was good therapy, relaxing, and family and friends could join together in this activity.

Knowing that her daughter would most likely not totally recover from her stroke, Joan felt thankful that Michelle had lived a very active life; lots of friends, traveling, piloting a plane, a good education.

Some people would ask Joan, "Why Michelle?" Joan would say, "I don't know." And she would think there was no point in dwelling on this question. She needed to remain positive. Each small improvement with Michelle's physical recovery would give Joan hope, for she knew these miniscule achievements were to indicate how well Michelle would do in the future. Doctors kept giving the family encouragement, yet remained realistic. Hospital staff fell in love with Michelle as she showed such determination through her struggle. Joan was immensely proud of her daughter.

Gordon was initially numbed by Michelle's medical misadventure. However, he eventually came to terms with her poor prognosis for the future. He found himself wavering between hope and miracles, reality and despair; "How is my bright, 25 year old daughter to have a life, a life back?" Gordon would try to be optimistic when telling people of Michelle's prognosis, but he was not so convinced within himself. He was a realist. Some would say he was pessimistic. But Gordon called it straight. He could not live in myths.

On the other hand, Gordon had to protect his family and friends from Michelle's true reality, especially Michelle herself and, of course, Cori. Their hope was for Michelle's return to something normal, or an outcome better than paralysis.

On top of Gordon's relief of witnessing signs that Michelle's memory and brain function were intact came his anguish with Michelle's difficulty in communicating her thoughts. Others were ecstatic at a mere finger movement from Michelle. For Gordon, this was encouraging, but he was impatient for more progress to happen. He felt, as time passed without recovery, more doubt in the possibility of that recovery.

So Gordon waited. With Michelle he offered encouragement, massaged her body, helped her exercise, brought her news from the outside world, and welcomed the marvelous stream of family, friends, well-wishers, cards, stuffies, and messages. He was truly humbled by this tremendous support. He no longer answered the questions of "Why a 25 year old?" He simply focused on how to help her out of it.

Because it was obvious Michelle's stay in the hospital would be very long term, Gordon had to make the decision of how he was going to juggle his family life at home in Kamloops with his need to be with his youngest daughter. There was the question of whether or not he and Joan should move to Victoria. Gordon and Joan had several discussions with their friends, and also Paul, about their agony. They really did not want to move away from their long-time home and finally opted to commute back and forth between Kamloops and Victoria. The times of their departures from the hospital for Kamloops were difficult. Gordon carried some guilt. He felt bad for Cori and also Michelle. He and Joan did not realize until much later how their absences caused resentment and anger with Cori. To them, Cori seemed strong. But she needed them much more than they realized. They didn't know.

• • •

Over ten years later, Cori spoke about her feelings at that time. "Yes, I had to deal with them coming and going and I felt they were going home more than coming to Victoria. I still had work and yet I felt that someone should be with Michelle as much as possible because then we could help move limbs and keep her limber and using her muscles and that could have been done every morning and afternoon, but I could only visit late afternoon/evening and didn't want to spend all that time moving her limbs. I felt there were many things to continue to do for her and with her and I couldn't do it all by myself. I felt they were the parents and should be doing all they could for her – even like moving to Victoria to be there for her."

• • •

Michelle was definitely trying to communicate her desire for certain things. She would motion her head and eyes towards the feeding machine when she was hungry. She nodded her head to indicate "yes." She would motion her eyes to the doorway to let others know there was a nurse entering the room. It was clear that Michelle was developing her communication skills.

Joan and Gordon arrived one day from Kamloops and filled Michelle in on their week away. When they described seeing three pods of killer whales, over twenty of them, in Active Pass, Michelle listened intently, although she still seemed somewhat confused.

Mom and dad took Michelle outside into the sunshine for about an hour. Later in the day a nurse reported Michelle had been crying. Why? When Joan and Gordon took Michelle outside the next day and showed her their vehicle and the new storage bin they had for her stuff, tears once again came. "Michelle had quite a cry... Anyways, both mom and Michelle had tears!"

The family was noticing some encouraging movements and changes with Michelle. She could move her tongue back and forth and up and down. She could hold up her head for over an hour. Sometimes she would make sounds when inhaling, testing her vocal chords. She could move her head and neck and right hand. Swallowing was much easier for her now. And something wonderful happened; Michelle called out "mom" with her voice. Hurray!!

The medical people were now about to allow Michelle to go out of the hospital for a few hours at a time - to the beach, or a matinee, or the IMAX. A custom cab would have to be reserved and the excursion would have to be approved by Dr. Martin. Michelle would have to wear a soft collar for her neck. Michelle could go out, between 11am and 1 pm, whenever she wished. It was a milestone.

It was Michelle's one hundredth day in the hospital. Such a huge number for a rather uneventful day. The routine was the same. The nurses were the same. Visitors came and went, as per usual.

Michelle was unaware of the plan Cori was making. Cori was eager to take her sister somewhere fun. When Cori finally felt the plans for the outing were achievable, she asked Michelle if she was "cleared for takeoff." Gordon, however, was not sure Michelle was ready for this kind of excitement. It was clear that Cori and her father had different views on what was best for Michelle.

• • •

Now that Michelle was moving her head back and forth, even on the pillow, she was given a call bell that was placed under her ear. This new gadget would give Michelle the freedom of asking for assistance rather than just waiting helplessly for someone to finally come to her room. Nursing staff also supplied Michelle with a neck collar and neck pillow for support while in the wheelchair. Michelle found this helpful. Another addition to assist in Michelle's daily life was a switch to turn the radio on and off, and Michelle made a great effort in learning how to use it.

When Cori visited her one evening she discovered, through a note from a friend, Kristy, that Michelle had lifted her left shoulder three times, as if to reach across her body for something. Cori also found out from Adele, another of Michelle's friends, that Michelle squeezed with her right hand. Cori seemed shocked with this information. Was Michelle's strength in her right hand rather than her left? Cori would have to watch for that. In the meantime, Cori watered Michelle's plants, had a catch-up talk with her, and observed her use of both her head signalers.

Every once in a while there would be a note in Michelle's diary from Scott. He would tell her he hoped she was feeling better and would pass on lots and lots of love. Once again, Scott's presence would be felt in his creative thought in writing future messages for Michelle many months ago.

There was disappointing news. Cathy, the occupational therapist, informed Cori that HandyDART could not take a Broda chair safely. HandyDART is a transportation service for persons who have a severe enough disability that the person is unable to use conventional transit service without assistance. Cathy was attempting to get an acceptable chair, but could not put the plans together in time for Cori's hopeful outing on Thursday. When Michelle was told of this she was clearly upset.

Cori arrived in the late afternoon one day to find Michelle on the verge of tears. Michelle was staring out the window, the radio was on, but the head clicker, the one that operated the radio, wasn't near Michelle's head. Cori believed her sister was frustrated, and talked to Michelle about her mood. Michelle indicated she was angry with the nurses. Cori didn't know how long Michelle had been left alone to fend for herself; she did know that she was Michelle's first visitor that day. Cori wrote, "She must get used to this."

That same evening one of the nurses, Patti, was getting Michelle ready for bed. Pattie was dancing to Spirit of the West and telling Michelle of her fun filled weekend. Michelle was nodding her head to the discussion. When Patti asked Michelle if she was warm enough, Michelle nodded her head. Patti was very excited with Michelle's new ability.

When Tammi visited Michelle the next day, she noticed "real good head movements." Tammi had shown Michelle some posters.

And she could tell that Michelle was trying to say something. Maybe Michelle was trying to say "thank you."

It had been three months since Michelle had been outside of the hospital environment; three months since she had stood on two legs, driven her sister's truck, joined friends at a local bar, or spoken a simple hello. Cathy, the occupational therapist was working very hard trying to obtain an available wheelchair for Michelle. Soon, Michelle would venture out.

Chapter 18

Cori was a very organized person. She would even say "super organized". She used a calendar for everything, would write notes on what to do most days, "almost anally so, like OCD sometimes." Everything would have its place in a room, and if someone moved it out of place, Cori would put it back. Clean and neat is how she liked it. "Or fake clean…you know, dusting superficially, vacuuming, but not to actual corners or spots that people can't see." And Cori realized that Michelle liked this too. She seemed to appreciate when Cori would clean up her room and put things where they should be, quickly and efficiently.

When Cori thought of those first weeks of dealing with Michelle's emergency, it was like a bad dream. There was so much about those days that was lost to her memory forever, as if nature had taken over and spared her many of the awful details. Cori didn't even recall where she'd slept that first night. Was it in the lobby at ICU? Did she sleep on the couch? She couldn't remember. She didn't even have a recollection of sleeping in her own bed for those first few months.

Crying came later. She would cry by herself in her bed, in her room. Or there would be tears shed whenever she related the story to others, as when she first told Tammi; and when she first saw her parents at the hospital. There were complete breakdowns, where Cori would let out her frustrations with the medical system. And, yes, there was that nagging disappointment with her parents' decision to remain living in Kamloops.

• • •

It was September. Gordon and Joan and Paul were there from Kamloops for a visit with Michelle. They took her outside in her wheelchair. It was raining. Paul and Gordon wheeled her up and down the trail between the intermittent showers. Michelle enjoyed the sound, sight, smell and feel of the rain. She was excited about her anticipated outing with Cori, yet it did frighten her. She had been sheltered from real life for so many months. Michelle confessed, "Yes of course I knew I didn't like being there but I knew I couldn't handle 'the real world' anymore."

That evening Joan and Gordon were aware that Michelle was in pain. Her back and legs were kinked. They tried to reposition her and, when the nurse arrived, Michelle was moved and readied for the night. Gordon read to Michelle from the book "Small Miracles" along with a couple of pages of "Far Side."

Family was still noticing slight improvements over time. Paul noted that Michelle gave one squeeze with her left hand and was able to regularly squeeze with her right hand. And he could tell that Michelle was trying to talk and was making some tones with her voice. Mom and dad even played catch with Michelle with a soft yellow ball that Gordon would place in her right hand and Michelle would let drop into her mom's hand.

Happy tears were shed the next day when Michelle kept moving her lips and finally said "Happy…" This was meant to be a Happy Birthday wish to her mom. Michelle then said in a loud whisper "I Love You." Both Joan and Michelle had another happy cry. It was a joyful evening.

Joan's birthday was on September 9, the one hundred and fourteenth day of Michelle's seemingly permanent residence at the hospital. They all went, except Michelle, to Romeo's for dinner. It was a gathering of eight of Joan's family and friends. After dinner they went to Grandma's for cake and ice cream. About 10 p.m. that night Joan and Gordon went back to the hospital for a quick visit with Michelle. They told her all about the evening. It was something in which Michelle would usually have been involved, this birthday celebration. It was happy. It was sad.

The next day Joan and Gordon left for Kamloops where they would stay for two weeks.

Cathy, the occupational therapist, finally acquired a new wheelchair for Michelle. It was the latest technology. Michelle sat up in the new chair for an hour. The chair was tilted at a 45 degree angle, so Michelle's head was supported by the headrest. According to Cathy, the chair would cost $4,000.00 and was on loan to Michelle for one week for assessment purposes. Funding for this chair would definitely be an issue. Who would pay for this? Michelle would also need power mobility once she could manage the controls. Cathy was hopeful that Michelle would soon be able to go on an excursion.

A brief note in Michelle's diary from one of the nurses mentioned Michelle's happiness at successfully using the bedpan.

The following day Tammi came in to shave Michelle's legs. They had some laughs. But, at 2 p.m., after Tammi had left, one of the nurses noticed Michelle crying. The nurse turned Michelle and repositioned her in the bed, which seemed to settle Michelle down. The nurse questioned what the problem could have been. Upset? Discomfort? Spasm? Gordon and Joan called from Kamloops to see how she was doing. Did that lift her spirits? Later on Cori came by with her boyfriend, Javier, and was very impressed with Michelle's new chair. She definitely planned on taking Michelle out, somewhere.

Michelle was trying very hard to talk. Cori thought Michelle looked tense when she tried, but Michelle insisted that she wasn't. It seemed to Cori that Michelle had more of her own sound now when she laughed. Even though the practice sessions with Michelle's speech, to Cori, could "freak someone out", Cori believed they were very beneficial to Michelle. And Cori noticed that Michelle moved various parts of her body much more when she was attempting to vocalize.

It was Saturday, and the time had finally arrived for Michelle to explore the real world. She was carefully loaded into the HandyDART and they all went to Beacon Hill Park. Michelle was smiling and laughing all the time. She recognized the downtown area. When they met Tammi at the petting zoo, they ventured through the zoo and met Kira, a one week old goat that sat on Michelle's lap. Little Kira clearly enjoyed all the petting. Michelle, always looking in the air for planes, saw a helicopter. It was a two hour outing. Michelle was physically tired; her neck and head hurt a bit, but she loved her adventure and wanted to do it as often as possible.

• • •

At eighteen years of age, in the summer of 1992, Michelle travelled to Europe with her mom and dad and, her brother, Paul. Cori had just recently been on a similar trip and remained home to work. It was clear from comments Michelle made in her diary that she was excited to be travelling, yet very much missed her social life with her friends back in Canada.

One of Michelle's greatest entertainments throughout her trip was all the cute guys, beginning with the "young lookers" that served as flight attendants on the plane trip. Young Michelle wrote that they were gorgeous.

When the family arrived in Frankfurt, Germany they briefly stayed with Gordon's brother, Ron, and his wife, Verna who were now living in Germany. Ron worked for a company that stationed him in Germany for a two year period. After a day or so, the Brittons rented a VW Passat station-wagon and headed out on the *Autobahn*. Michelle described the slow cars travelling at about 100 kilometers per hour while the fast cars were doing about 200. She was thrilled. But Michelle was not impressed with her visit to the Museum of

Roman Ruins because all of the written explanations of the ruins were in German. She grew bored with it all. She did, however, enjoy the Dome Cathedral with its 509 steps to the top. And Michelle couldn't help but notice the "good looking guys around." She thought it would be "neat" to come back to this area with a friend when she could "do whatever you felt like doing."

When she went up for her second visit to the top of the Eiffel Tower her comment was simply "I love it." All the things to see in Paris were somewhat entertaining for Michelle, but what she enjoyed most was watching the people. She found them so interesting. She enjoyed her encounter with a man selling postcards and was delighted when he told her mother that Michelle was beautiful.

The Louvre was a huge disappointment to Michelle. "Remind me to never to back," she wrote in huge block letters in her diary. She was frustrated by the immense volume of artwork on display that, to her, looked all the same. But the day wasn't a total waste. Later on, in a café, the waiter playfully flirted with Michelle, calling her "sweet one" and "darling." She clearly enjoyed the attention.

Even though Michelle "loved" being in Europe, she couldn't stop thinking about home. She would see people in Europe who would remind her of her friends in Kamloops. She wondered what Wes and Jon were doing. Michelle and Wes were at an impasse, and not really a couple anymore. She wondered if Wes was seeing Lisa, and Michelle couldn't quite figure out if Wes seeing Lisa was something good or not. Things had not been good with Wes. The two of them seemed to be heading in different directions in their plans towards the future.

The last day in Paris involved the family's visit to the Paris Opera house. This impressed Michelle. She fantasised what it would be like to see one of the operas in this exciting place. They walked down to the Champs-Elysees and on to the Arc de Triumph. While her dad and Paul ventured up the arc, Michelle and her mom relaxed below. Once again, Michelle was happy to just sit and watch the people. It seemed to be her favourite pastime. And she was excited when a group of tourists asked her to join in the group picture. She had her picture taken beside "this great looking guy." She couldn't believe how people, on the Metro, kept staring at her. Several times Michelle was told that she was beautiful. Michelle thought that was funny. She seemed unaware of her unique attractiveness.

Michelle felt a bit dizzy that day. She thought that maybe she was just tired.

From Paris the family moved on to Fontainebleau. Michelle was beginning to tire, and she missed home "more and more." She missed her friends and Cori and showers and tap water and freedom and familiar language and relaxation. She was experiencing headaches and dizziness. Maybe it was the heat. The temperature had been over 30 degrees. Thoughts of Wes, Jon, Mark, and Manny were swimming around in her head all day. Michelle felt very tired.

That night she experienced a very disturbing dream about Wes. She had returned home from her European venture and he had totally ignored her and was flirting with another girl. Michelle thought about the dream most of the day. She wasn't sure if she was upset over Wes being interested in another girl or the fact he had ignored her. But she was certainly angry in the dream. During the day she sometimes felt like crying and asked herself "What's wrong with me?" In her diary that evening she ended her writing with, "I wish I were home."

The family travelled on to Switzerland. Michelle loved the beauty of the landscape, which was like a "Heidi" scene. But the long hours in the car were definitely beginning to tire her, and spending every hour of every day with her mom, dad, and brother was making her depressed and longing for her friends at home. She figured this was the reason she often felt like crying. She simply missed her personal social life.

The excursion up the Swiss Alps was a perfect day. The weather was beautiful. Michelle watched the "guys" hang gliding and parachuting. It took the family 5 ½ hours to take the gondola up the mountain and hike back down. Luckily, it did not start to rain until they made it back to their car. After dinner that evening, they made a trip to the laundry. "What a way to spend a Friday night," Michelle wrote.

Spending the night at a dairy farm bed and breakfast was one of the highlights of Michelle's vacation. She was thrilled with a tour through the barns to see the cows and horses. She wrote in her diary about a 14 kilometer tunnel they drove through. And she mentioned Wes and her relationship with him, how she missed him.

"The view was unbelievable" in Austria, but Michelle was not impressed with the Austrians. She found them to be abrupt and rude. At one point in her diary she said, "I hate Austrians, they're so rude and grumpy." Michelle wrote almost every day that she missed her friends and wished she were home. One day her frustration was illustrated by the comment, "I need to get away…I miss people my own age really bad…I need to socialize…Aargh!"

Part of the tour was a visit to Mozart's birthplace and a wonderful Sound of Music tour. At a beer garden Michelle's parents even allowed her to have half a beer. The next day they all went to the Deutsches Museum. Michelle was fascinated with the place and thought that every man should visit there with its abundance of planes, trains, automobiles and musical instruments. Later on they went to another beer garden and Michelle's dad bought her another beer, which Michelle said was "cool." The next day the destination was Heidelberg where Michelle had her third beer, something that was a very unique experience, drinking with her parents.

Finally, they were back at Ron and Verna's. Michelle was so relieved that she now had people around her who actually spoke English. Michelle and Paul spent quite a bit of time at the pool. There were four pools and a waterslide and huge diving boards. The weather was cool, but time at the pool was such a nice break from all the driving and visiting castles. It was also a refreshing break from being with her parents. And, of course there were lots of great looking guys around. Michelle especially liked the guys wearing "those great European Speedos."

She had an "awesome" day at the beach in Holland on the North Sea. She swam. She fought the waves. She tanned in the sun. She felt like a total beach bum, with sand in her eyes, hair, and bathing suit. And her face was burned. It was a very good day. The family saw Holland's canals and windmills and an "awesome sunset." When Michelle removed her bathing suit at the end of the day she found lots of sand and "even a sea shell."

The pool became a huge enjoyment for Michelle. She met two "babes" there, Gordon from Yugoslavia and Alberto from Italy. They all agreed, Michelle's cousin Kathy included, to meet at the Cathedral in Koln the next day. They walked around the old town by the river; then they went to a disco. Gordon and Michelle spent a little time dancing. She liked the way he danced. When they got too warm from the exertion, they snuggled up on a couch. They kissed. On the way back to the train they walked and talked and kissed some more. When the girls arrived at their train stop, Michelle's dad and aunt were waiting for them. The adults were "pretty worried." It was 1:30 in the morning.

Michelle and Kathy went to the pool for a few hours the next day, spending time with the boys. Gordon called Michelle later on that evening and asked everyone to come down to a fair. So they all joined up at the fair and had a great time. "It was crazy." The only down side to the day was Michelle's mother. Joan seemed unhappy with Michelle's adventurous ways with the boys. Michelle wrote, "I'm 18 for $%&# sakes. I know what I'm doing."

On their last evening in Europe everyone gathered at Ron and Verna's. Michelle insisted on having young Gordon over and there was confusion on what train station to pick him up. Consequently, Michelle's parents were not pleased with her inviting her "boyfriend" over and causing such trouble. Auntie Verna was a good peacemaker host, however, and they all had a nice but uncomfortable evening together. When Michelle's mom and dad dropped Gordon off at the train station, Michelle threw caution to the wind and hugged and kissed him. They exchanged addresses and she hoped he would write her.

It was the end of the holiday. But it was only the beginning of Michelle's obsession with seeing the world.

Chapter 19

It was the middle of September and, written in Michelle's diary, was a message from Scott, telling her he was sending her all of his love "right now at this very minute." It was such a wonderful idea that Scott had come up with, writing once in a while a happy note in her diary. Whenever a note was discovered, Cori would excitedly read it to Michelle. It would make Michelle smile or giggle. "It was so Scott."

Tammi remained a dutiful friend over the months. She regularly worked on Michelle's nails, remarking one day on how "So, so, so, so beautiful" Michelle's purple nails were with their blue decorations "on every nail."

Cori was always looking for those miniscule improvements in Michelle that would inspire Cori to have faith in her sister's future. When taken down to the gift store, Michelle was positioned by the window and moved her head from left to right "FULLY & WITHOUT MUCH ENERGY." Cori signed her diary notation with two exclamation marks and a big smiley face.

Cori had an incredible ability to deal with Michelle's struggle in a positive way: "Frustrations…I don't remember having too many. I knew it was a long, slow road, so I wasn't wishing to rush it. I always had hope. Me and my friends would try all sorts of things – classical music to stimulate the brain, bringing a guitarist in to play specially for Michelle, reading books out loud to her, pushing the limits (like taking her around the hospital as soon as she could). Bad doctors…I don't believe I ever thought they were bad at all. There were definitely favourite nurses – the ones who took a moment to be human and joke with Michelle or take some time to get to know her or us – they were truly amazing folk. It was always nice to come see Michelle and see a nurse we know and chit-chat with them a moment. Felt more like a home than a hospital. Tired…I don't remember feeling tired, nope. I may have been tired from working, but my first thought was always how Michelle always lifted me up – I always left Michelle that night feeling revived, at peace, laughing about something we joked about or how it was great to see her smile. I enjoyed my visits at the hospital with my sister, and family or friends. I think I saw more friends that first six months than I ever had. It was nice that way. I also don't think I was depressed; I found myself living for Michelle – if she were going to fight and be happy in the hospital, then so was I – keep positive, keeping hope alive, etc. I don't remember being depressed at all."

There were a few daily complications in Michelle's life. Her remote control for her radio was not working. Paul thought it needed to be re-charged, however, the occupational therapist informed him that the remote was on an infra-red system. These gadgets were hi-tech and certainly challenged everyone's technical knowledge. And Michelle's trial wheelchair had to be returned, so she was back in her Broda chair. There were to be discussions between the therapists and the family about how Michelle could purchase the new chair. It now appeared that the quality of Michelle's life would be determined by her financial status.

The next gadget offered by "the system" was an augmentative communication device. This machine was operated by Michelle looking at 8 squares, each of them relaying a common message she would like to use. The messages would be recorded by Cori.

Therapists were now trying to feed Michelle by mouth, using a thick liquid that would not choke her. Michelle's constant battle with thrush often hindered the progress. Therapists hoped that doctors would give the go ahead with oral feeding on a regular basis.

To Michelle's excitement, Scott managed to catch a flight on a Challenger airplane from Nova Scotia to Comox. He made his way south on Vancouver Island to Victoria and visited for a couple of hours. He stayed overnight at Paul's place and visited her on and off for most of the next day. He took her outside to see the bunnies. They joked and laughed, and Michelle was even trying to kick him, in fun. Scott thought her improvements were incredible, and was amazed that she was now so active. He also managed to communicate with her using a letter board. It was a learning process for him. The board contained all the letters of the alphabet on a grid. Michelle would blink the appropriate number of times to move across the board. She would then pause for a second and blink the appropriate number of times to move down the board. It was slow. Michelle became very economical with her words. But they were talking. Scott was thrilled with her responsiveness.

At the end of his visit Scott wrote, "Physio was working with Michelle. I sat in and watched. For a moment, Shell got frustrated and started to cry; before long she was laughing again. We worked with the letter board a bit. Bye Shelley. Lots of love. See you soon. Scott."

HandyDART was now willing to take Michelle in her Broda chair. She no longer had to wait for her new wheelchair to go on outings, although it was clear the newer chair would be much better for her in the future. Cori and her parents took Michelle out the very next day. In preparation for the outing, a collar was put around Michelle's neck to provide support in the moving vehicle. It became instantly apparent that Michelle was "very uncomfortable" with the collar when she began crying. So they decided not to use it. Instead, they tilted Michelle back in her chair and leaned her head on a support in the chair. It was fine. They went to Beacon Hill Park and strolled around in the sunshine, taking in the beauty of the gardens and ponds. Michelle enjoyed her outing but she was extremely conscious of being disabled in public. The real reason she did not want the collar put on was: "The collar wasn't painful but I already felt like a freak so that was worse and it made it difficult to look around." At the end of the day, she appeared happy and relaxed.

Gordon and Joan noted how strong Michelle's legs were becoming. She was able during exercises to push out each leg and bend it at the knee. They mentioned they were very excited to see Michelle's progress on this visit and commented on what a wonderful improvement in only four months. They wondered, at this rate, how much better she would be in eight months. It was "really encouraging." At this time, they were returning home to Kamloops and planning an extended long weekend visit with Michelle for Thanksgiving. They believed they had "lots to give thanks for!"

Another visitor Michelle spent time with was Olivia, a student volunteer. She had been to Africa and brought in pictures she had taken of elephants. Cori left Olivia a note explaining that Michelle had travelled to New Zealand and Australia and had spent 5 months in Banff. This was Cori's way of trying to show others the real Michelle, the well-educated, well-travelled Michelle.

There were several therapists working with Michelle. They would get Michelle to try sucking and blowing with a straw; and relaxing and opening her hands. They had meetings with her parents and discussed various types of therapies and how these therapies worked. Michelle's physical improvements were monitored and her future move to the GF Strong Rehabilitation Hospital in Vancouver was considered. But it was decided that Michelle was not quite ready physically for this move. Joan and Gordon spoke with Sandy Fulton, Michelle's social worker, about a new wheelchair. They filled out some application forms.

It was so nice that Michelle was finally getting out of the hospital. The entire family spent a day with her at Willows Beach. It was a bright, sunny, calm, fresh morning as they headed outdoors. Joan and Michelle rode together in the HandyDART bus. Tammi, Cori, Kristy and Javier met them there at the beach. Paul and Gordon came a bit later. A gathering of family and friends, outside the hospital, was a welcome experience for Michelle. She then joined the family at Grandma Britton's apartment on Thanksgiving Day. Michelle was dressed in a turtleneck and overalls, and "looked HOT," according to Cori's observation. It was also noted that Michelle was holding up her head quite well and was getting much stronger.

On the last day of Joan and Gordon's Thanksgiving visit with Michelle they sat with her in her hospital room, watching TV. Michelle was quite upset and was crying. Was she lonely? Frustrated? They thought she may have a leg cramp so they straightened her out on her back and massaged her legs. This seemed to help, but she still moaned. Joan tried to work with Michelle on the letter board to figure out Michelle's problem, but it became frustrating. Joan just couldn't get it. Michelle cried again. Joan agonized over her failure to help her daughter. It all seemed so unfair. In retrospect, Joan was glad that Michelle had tried things like flying an airplane, risky adventures that Joan often in the past had tried to stop Michelle from doing; out of a mother's love, and an instinct to protect. She was glad that Michelle had done a lot of living in her first 24 years.

Joan and Gordon wrote a goodbye note to Michelle before their return to Kamloops. "All our love, dear! You keep cheerful, optimistic, and practise things you know will help your progress!"

Therapists tried a control switch for Michelle to use for turning on and off the radio and TV. But Michelle had progressed to the point where she could control a switch with her ever strengthening right hand. And she definitely preferred this control. She was also beginning to read. Therapists would make the print large and would cover the lines above and below the text she was reading. She was enjoying this. And she was trying so hard to speak. Her top lip would quiver. But she could not control her lips or her tongue. And she could not produce enough air from her lungs to force out the words.

Good news. Funding for Michelle's new wheelchair purchase was approved. It was on order.

On Halloween, Michelle chose royal blue and grape colors for her finger nails. Some nurses painted her toenails orange. Michelle was able to suck on a sucker. There were lots of laughs.

Progress was being made on plans to transfer Michelle to GF Strong. The health care "team" for Michelle would provide Gord Manning, the Admissions Coordinator of GF Strong, with information needed for her approval for admission. She would be placed in GF Strong for a three week period of assessment. Michelle was happy about the move to GF Strong. She knew they could help her.

She now had a new control. It was a Kincontrol. She used her right hand, her fingers, to hit a knob to turn on the radio or call bell. She loved it! She was one step closer to her independence.

• • •

Michelle and Cori came up with some phrases for the augmentative communication device.

"No, but…"

"Yes, but…"

"Thank you very much"

"I don't know"

"I'm happy today"

"I'm in a bad mood"

"Hello"

"My hair needs undoing!"

It was interesting to see what was on the *important list* with Michelle. A woman's hair can take priority to almost everything.

With the alphabet board Michelle was now communicating her needs. She could complain if the TV was too loud. Or she could let someone know if she had any pain. Sometimes her left hip would hurt if she was lying on her left side. Now, she could let her parents know that. And now the nurses could be made aware of these types of problems.

There was a dinner party at Grandma Britton's. The partyers included Grandma, Cori, Javier, Paul, Jenn, Tammi, Joan, Gordon and, very special guest, Michelle. Everybody had a great time eating Chinese food and Spumante. Michelle even had a teaspoon of mint ice cream, and some chocolate ice cream later on in the afternoon. At the end of the day, Michelle did not want to back in to the hospital. So the family walked her around the hospital parking lot for a while. It was noted in Michelle's diary that she was comfortable in her wheelchair for 3 hours and 40 minutes.

The next day Michelle was very upset. Her parents were leaving for 3 weeks and the rest of her family, Cori and Paul, would be gone for a few days. Joan and Gordon suspected Michelle was frustrated, or possibly feeling bad that everyone was going away. Finally Michelle spelled out the word "USELESS."

In the morning, Jenn and Paul discovered that Michelle was fine. She had simply become frustrated with the letter board, nothing more. Jenn and Paul guessed that Michelle may have been working with the board for too extended a time, especially because it had been late at night and Michelle may have been over tired from the long day. Her parents had felt really bad leaving Michelle when "she had such a downer."

There was a TV for Michelle in her room that she could now control with her KinControl. She could change the channels and turn the volume up and down. But this would only work for Michelle if it was hooked up properly. Tammi tried to do this one day, but she couldn't figure it out. Michelle laughed at her friend and Tammi wrote "someone with more brains could do it for her. Ha! Ha! Sorry."

An example of the technical complication with the seemingly easy task of hooking up a TV was described by Michelle's occupational therapist, Cathy: "KinControl now wired to TV and converter, however, awaiting cable adaptor as cable hook-up not possible until Biomedical engineers link adaptor. Contact made but adaptor cable may need to be built in Biomed. Sorry about delay but we ARE working on TV control." Technology was to become a very important part of Michelle's daily life, her link to the world.

G.F. Strong people assessed Michelle and decided she may move to their rehab in the New Year. Michelle was becoming impatient with her rehabilitation. She wanted more controls hooked up so she could begin working with them. She and Cori were getting the hang of communicating with the alphabet board and were both excited with this improvement in their lives. The only setback for Michelle was the fatigue she experienced when using the TV control. Each movement took all her strength and was overwhelmingly tiring. She would often be forced to return to the old methods for a while until her energy returned.

Michelle's new wheelchair had arrived at the supplier and was being assembled. Cori met with a few of the "team" members and was informed that Michelle was not swallowing good enough to have food orally. When the feeding tube that was now going into her stomach wore out, it would be replaced with a button so that the new tube could be removed between feedings. This would eliminate a tube being constantly extending from her body. A tube would now only be used during feeding times. Cori was also informed that there was a bed ready for Michelle at the Gorge Road Hospital. There would be a three week wait for a room in the Young Adult area. Cori was told there would be "NO LONG TERM REHAB."

Gorge Road Hospital is a facility located in the Gorge neighbourhood and is close to a medium-sized mall, grocery store, and small restaurants. The hospital was built in 1973. Residential services are provided on two floors of the four floor building. The building is adjacent to the Gorge waterway with the rear of the building facing the water. There is a grassy knoll area behind the building, as well, for residents to enjoy and walk about. Each floor of the hospital has an outdoor recreation area equipped with patio furniture and a BBQ. A hair salon is operated on the first floor. Both floors have resident lounges.

This did not seem to be the appropriate facility for Michelle. It appeared there would be no rehabilitation program within the hospital. This hospital was a "Complex Care" facility that offered support for people requiring 24-hour care. The hospital did not advertise that it offered a rehabilitation program. In fact, all it boasted were various activities such as "exercise groups, arts and crafts, bingo, entertainment groups and special events." The move to this facility would be a stressful event for Michelle. Cori informed her sister, thinking it would be better for her to hear this news from a member of the family. Michelle did not seem overly upset with this upcoming change.

In the meantime, Heather, one of the occupational therapists noted that family needed to work aggressively with Michelle's swallowing. When Heather fed Michelle some Chocolate Boost, she was impressed by Michelle's ability to swallow. Heather was quite sure Michelle could improve this ability, and Heather wrote, "It is very important to Shell to eat normally."

The University of Victoria granted Michelle her degree, seeing she had been so close to finishing her studies before her stroke happened. On November 26, 1999, the nurses put on a graduation party for Michelle. She was all fixed up, nice hair and make-up, looking "absolutely marvellous." The family attended. There was music. There was laughter. There were tears. Michelle was very touched. She said, "I am usually so tough!"

The following day Cori picked Michelle up from the hospital. Once again Michelle had her hair all fixed up and make-up on. She was "very beautiful." Cori and Tracey, a nurse, took Michelle to the university and helped Michelle into her cap, gown, and shoes. Michelle and her entourage went through the ceremonies "without a hitch." When Michelle was wheeled across the stage, EVERYONE applauded. A photographer from the local newspaper took her picture. At the end of the day Michelle was tired. The event of her graduation was bittersweet. It was wonderful that all of her hard work had finally paid off and she was now finished with her studies. She was sad, though, with the idea that she would most likely lose touch with the many friendships she had developed over the years in university. And she still did not know what type of career she would choose. At this point in her life, she wondered if there would be anything at all in her future.

Her parents wrote, "We are so proud of you! Congratulations!"

• • •

Financial assistance for Michelle from the government would be an ongoing struggle. Sandy Fulton comments on this aspect of living with a disability. "Funding for the wheelchair came from the ministry, social services. I filled in all the forms. I think we must have applied for income assistance because Michelle had no income, so we would have applied for disability level 2, I think it was called at that time. If you were at level 2 you would get more money than if you were just a single woman living on your own with no children. The difference is probably about $450.00 a month. And because she's a disabled person she has some funding available for a wheelchair and specialized equipment. The disability application is about 23 pages long and if you don't dot every 'I' and cross every 'T', they'll shoot it back to you. We had a big whoop-d-do on the unit when her chair came. I think we got a cake for her."

Chapter 20

Adele Colistro was Michelle's childhood friend. The two girls grew up as neighbours, schoolmates, friends and "sometimes rivals." Michelle, in Adele's mind, was easy to like and easy to talk to. Adele loved her infectious laugh. Adele also thought her friend had a kind heart.

There was a close family connection with the two girls. Their mothers were good friends. Adele's dad had been their teacher. And Adele's sister was friends with Michelle's brother, Paul.

Michelle was a part of Adele's everyday life. They were both bright and intelligent, always achieving top grades in school. The girls shared lots of memories. There were birthday parties, baking cookies, summer days riding their bikes, and climbing onto to roof of her backyard shed to talk. Adele enjoyed listening to her friend practice piano or watching her tap dance routine to Zippidy-do-da. They most often walked to school together. They most often went together trick or treating on Halloween, and would join a neighbourhood party for hot chocolate and fireworks.

One time, Michelle wanted to bleach her new jeans. Adele helped her carefully place the jeans in the washing machine. Acid-wash jeans were the in thing, and Michelle just had to do this. It was a fun experiment, but her mom was "pretty mad" with Michelle's risky behaviour.

Michelle was the more outgoing of the two. Adele was not nearly as confident. It was likely because of her friendship with Michelle that Adele participated in Brownies and, later on,

Explorers. They went to summer camp at their church's Camp Grafton as youngsters, and eventually became camp leaders. Adele's family always joined the group at Wallaper Lake every year for some outdoor winter fun.

Like most close friends, the girls had occasional disagreements, but these were soon forgotten. Adele was the one who jumped off the teeter totter at the school playground and sent Michelle falling to the ground, breaking her arm. Adele felt really bad. But she soon became jealous when Michelle came to school with her cast for everyone to sign, obviously quite thrilled with the attention.

As the two girls grew older into their teens, they developed different interests and hung out with different groups of friends. They didn't spend nearly as much time together. Their friendship, however, was well established and they would still do the odd thing together. The girls convinced their parents to allow them, along with Cori, to travel to France for two weeks. It was like old times as Adele and Michelle paired up on bus trips, hotel rooms and on all of the excursions.

The two young women did not keep in touch regularly as they moved on to college and university. Their parents would pass on to the girls updates on what the other was doing. They would see each other briefly on holidays and it was always easy for them to catch up where they had left off.

Adele was attending medical school at the University of British Columbia when she heard from her mother of Michelle's stroke. It was ironic that Adele was presently rotating through the Internal Medicine department at University Hospital and seeing stroke patients on a daily basis. So, it was not that she had absolutely no idea of what was happening to Michelle. Initially, Adele tried to downplay in her mind the seriousness of Michelle's medical prognosis. She would think, "After all, Michelle is young, healthy and vibrant." Adele told herself that Michelle would get through the acute period, do a bit of rehab, and recover and carry on. But, within a few weeks, the terrible reality of Michelle's condition set in. Adele knew it was not good.

The first time Adele visited Michelle after her stroke, Michelle was still in the hospital in Victoria. Adele and her boyfriend, Rob, took the ferry to Vancouver Island for the weekend with the intent to visit Michelle. "I was well prepared for the medical aspects of Michelle's condition and thought I would handle the situation well, but it is a very different experience when it is your friend and not your patient that is lying in that hospital bed."

The actual visit with Michelle was a blur for Adele. Michelle's parents acted as interpreters as Michelle spelled out words with a slow, laborious process of selecting the letters by row and column on a board and looking up with her eyes for 'yes' as her visitors tried to guess the right letter/word/phrase to speed up the process. Adele tried her best to make small talk and keep the conversation light and upbeat. She desperately tried to convince herself that there was still hope for progress and medical improvement and maybe even the miracle of complete recovery. Yet, she knew that would be impossible.

Adele and Rob left the hospital room and made it as far as the elevators before she broke down and sobbed.

• • •

The time finally came for Michelle to move on. Her stay at VGH had come to an end. It was no longer possible for the hospital to care for such a long term patient. Michelle was leaving everything familiar to her: her comfortable room that became her home, the daily routine she had grown so accustomed to; and the people. Nurses and therapists had become her friends. She knew she would probably never see them again. It was heartbreaking.

That first day in her new home at Gorge Road Hospital was both scary and exciting. Even though her family was right there with her, Michelle felt so alone. "I cried all day."

Tammi visited Michelle in her new room. She realized it was a huge change. She knew Michelle was not very happy and did her best to cheer her up. She moved things around in the room according to Michelle's instructions, helping her out as best she could. Paul came in and adjusted Michelle's head to a more comfortable position. Cori and Javier dropped by and chatted with Michelle about various things. They also met another patient, Wayne, who came by and introduced himself. He seemed like a great guy. He mentioned he had been at Gorge for 20 years. Cori didn't think Michelle had heard that comment. Maybe it was a good thing. Would that kind of information upset her?

Mike was Michelle's new physiotherapist, or PT, for short. He was already giving her homework. She was required to do ten chin tucks, to be performed slowly with a small hold at the end of the motion, three times a day. Allison was Michelle's new Occupational Therapist. The simple description of an OT is: one who helps the disabled person acquire the needed skills for the job of living. Allison helped set up all of Michelle's controls. The Kincontrol had the options of using it for the radio or for a call bell to the nurses. Michelle was using a switch they called a "jellybean switch" with her right hand. She was also set up with a "pad switch" that served as a call bell when Michelle was in bed.

Tammi came in the following morning and took Michelle outside for a walk. It was different here, much more hilly, and the sidewalks were very bumpy. She said that she and Michelle had a "4x4 experience". They sat down on the grass above the water. It was a bit breezy, but it was good to get outside.

Cori was pleased to find out that nurses had set up a machine to play videos and Michelle was busy watching them every night. So far, Michelle was receiving TV cable for free.

Paul spent a few hours with Michelle and was thrilled when she whispered his name. He even double checked to make sure she could really do it, and she said it again. He also observed that she was dancing with her fingers. Michelle was content.

Mike, her PT, wrote in Michelle's diary that she had tone in both hands and could turn her right hand palm up more easily. He mentioned how important it was to keep her fingers out straight.

Joan and Gordon arrived and found their daughter all settled in. They talked with Michelle and got caught up. They were excited. This was progress.

One day in mid-December the family took Michelle on an outing to Cori's place. Michelle ate some ice cream and very much enjoyed it. Then she sucked on a dill pickle, but accidently swallowed it. Everyone panicked. They didn't know if she had sucked it into her stomach or her lungs. They called 911. The ambulance fellows came and checked her lungs and pulse and blood pressure. She seemed okay. What a relief. HandyDART came to transport her back to the hospital and it was about 8:30 in the evening when she arrived. It was a long, stressful day. She was exhausted.

A meeting was to take place the following day with the "team" from GF Strong Rehabilitation Centre. This was the place where Michelle and her family knew her real recovery would take place.

• • •

The meaning of "tertiary": 1: Third in point of time, number, degree, etc.

GF Strong is a tertiary care facility specializing in rehabilitation services. The organization provides inpatient, outpatient, and outreach services to adolescents and adults throughout British Columbia and the Yukon.

Following World War II, there was a great need for the rehabilitation of disabled veterans. At that time, people with disabilities had to leave the province for their rehabilitation.

Dr. George Frederick Strong, a Vancouver internist, became one of the prime movers in the drive to establish a rehabilitation facility in British Columbia, after his daughter sustained a spinal cord injury. He joined forces with the Western Division of the Paraplegic Association through Mr. Ed Desjardins, a veteran who had become quadriplegic during the war. Mr. "D", as he was affectionately called, worked as the Director of the GF Strong Rehabilitation Centre for over 40 years and as a consultant until his death in 1998.

The meeting would involve advocating for Michelle. She needed more rehab. She needed to be in a more home-like environment for living. There were so many things to consider. Admission to GF Strong involved a long list of requirements. Referrals had to be made by a physician, and her most recent medical history and consultations were to be provided. Michelle's latest results of medical diagnostic tests were needed.

The list of GF Strong rehabilitation admission criteria was long. The applicant would need to have sustained significant loss of function as a result of brain injury, spinal cord injury, stroke or other disabling condition or disease process. There would have to be limitations in functional areas such as "mobility/motor, ADL (Activities of Daily Living), home/community management, respiratory, bowel/bladder control, cognition, swallowing and communication.

There was no question as to Michelle's meeting those requirements. Her loss of function included all of these areas. The cause of her condition was also completely acceptable to the rehabilitation centre. What would be of concern, however, was the next thing on the list of GF Strong: "(The applicant) has demonstrated rehabilitation potential with expectation for clinical/functional improvement and has identifiable rehabilitation goals."

This was the reason the "team" from GF Strong spent a full day with Michelle. They were assessing her ability and determination for improvement. The "team" was testing Michelle for the next requirement on the GF Strong list. "Able to follow visual/verbal commands and demonstrates a willingness/ability to actively participate and learn."

It was evident that Michelle was determined. Any person who knew Michelle would attest to her strong will and her desire to make a better life for herself. She was not the type of person to sit back and accept her condition without a good fight.

Michelle also qualified for other requirements. A patient of GF Strong was to need 24-hour nursing availability to assist with daily activities. A patient also required "physician assessment/oversight, program coordination, and medical specialty services, at a minimum of 3 times per week, based on clinical stability." The need for specialized therapeutic skills and equipment was another expectation for admission.

Michelle would have to be able to sit supported for at least one hour per day. Her need for therapy involving 2 or more disciplines such as Physical Therapy, Occupational Therapy or Speech Therapy was another requirement. She would have to show the ability to tolerate 3 hours of therapy per day, 5 days per week.

There were many other considerations for a patient's admission to GF Strong. These involved such things as clinical stability of the patient, and making certain that tube feedings would not interfere with physical therapy. It was a very structured and detailed application.

• • •

Michelle's new living quarters were being slowly set up to make her life as easy as possible. Her TV was working, and Michelle had a new control board allowing her to change the volume or channel with the touch of a finger. Another new thing for her was a computerized alphabet board where she could type messages. This new system also stored a variety of commonly used messages that Michelle could display with quickness and ease.

Michelle thought Mike was an attractive guy, maybe in his 30's. According to Michelle, it was commonly believed that most attractive men in Victoria were gay. This is what she thought of Mike. But she didn't know for sure. She thought he was great; so cheerful and positive. He would take her upstairs to the rehab room three times a week. This room had all kinds of physio "toys" like "plinth" beds, a tilt table, balls, exercise bikes and foam. Sometimes Mike would get help strap Michelle onto the tilt table. This is a padded board with straps across the knees, hips and chest. It tilts up until the person is more or less standing. Michelle was worked up to about 80 degrees. It really wasn't a natural standing position. It was explained to Michelle that this exercise would work different muscles in her body in different ways.

Positioning Michelle in a sitting position on the plinth was one more exercise to help strengthen her muscles. A plinth is a covered, matted flatbed where Michelle was most often laid down to stretch her limbs. But another exercise was to sit her upright on the edge with one person behind her and another person in front of her. This was a common position used to stimulate and strengthen the body core.

The age of increasingly complex technology would be of great assistance to Michelle. Although sometimes simple adjustments to the "techno" world would suffice, like when Allison, one of the OTs, mounted the remote control on a Kleenex box "so it would reach the TV more easily." Michelle was now using various machines. But there was a lot to remember. The switch to her Kincontrol needed to be plugged into the side of another machine. And that machine needed to be set up on the overhead table to allow Michelle to see it. It was also very important for her equipment to be plugged in "at the bedside by the bathroom" in order for the battery to charge. If this was not done, Michelle would lose her programming. The quality of Michelle's life definitely depended on the proper operation of her computerized equipment and the consistency of staff to keep it working.

Mike noted in Michelle's diary that she needed encouragement to keep her fingers straight. Seeing that she could now move her right hand on to and off of her button to operate her Kincontrol, it would be good for her hand if she tried to use the first knuckles of her fingers rather than using her wrist.

Wayne, Michelle's new skinny red-headed neighbour, was quite the character. He was quadriplegic. She wasn't sure how he had wound up that way, maybe a car accident. He maintained a very good sense of humour. But Michelle didn't really like him. He played hard, often going out drinking and smoking pot. A few times his wheelchair was taken away because he came home drunk. Michelle found it hard to tolerate "such habits and lack of respect of life."

Once again, Christmas had arrived. The family gathered at Cori's apartment. Cori brought Michelle over by HandyDART. They all had crackers, wine and a full dinner along with Grandma Britton's Christmas pudding. Gifts were exchanged. Then Cori returned Michelle to Gorge Road and wrote in her diary, "Great Day!"

Also written in Michelle's diary was a beautiful message from Scott. At the top left corner of the page he had drawn a holly leaf. In bold artistic lettering his message was "Merry Christmas Shelly, Love Scott." His drawing of a goofy face, the same one he drew in all of her messages, was at the bottom left of the message. In smaller lettering he wrote, "Smile Buddy." At the bottom right he drew a cute little picture of Rudolf with his sparkling nose. He wrote, "Rudolf Loves You Too."

• • •

After Michelle left VGH and moved to Gorge Road, Sandy Fulton was no longer required to have any contact with her. Sandy's job was to deal with patients at Victoria General and, when they moved on, Sandy's job was done.

Sandy did her best while Michelle was in the hospital to have her taken in by GF Strong. "We did teleconferences as well with GF Strong to make sure we were doing the right thing. GF Strong didn't feel that they had anything that they could offer that couldn't be done here in Victoria and that's when Michelle went to the Gorge. She went to the extended care at the Gorge. It was not what we had hoped for, for her. She went into extended care rather than into the rehab section. But the staff there fell in love with her and they got services for her that would not normally have been provided in extended care."

Chapter 21

There was certainly a degree of simplicity to Michelle's life now. People were helping her out by finding easy to use switches or buttons to control the TV or the radio. She was getting a new tray for her wheelchair. A bank account was set up for her so she could purchase items from the gift store or have her hair done by the hospital hairdresser. She could now pay for her own cable TV.

Other things were more difficult and complicated her life. How would she go the bathroom? Most people wouldn't even give it a thought. Michelle could control her bladder and hated to be left wet in her diaper. She began to make a noise when she needed to go. She relayed this information to Cori who was interested in Michelle's efforts and thought they should "work on this." But physio was Michelle's hugest task. Trying to move her head or her neck, or lift her shoulder or arm. These small movements would deplete her last bit of energy.

There were some good times now. Tammi and Cori would take Michelle out once in a while to the mall and they would shop around, or go somewhere for ice cream, Michelle's favorite. They would learn from this experience how other people viewed Michelle's condition. Tammi admitted she was once one of those people who were afraid of dealing with the disabled. In the past, when she would see someone with an uncontrollable body, in a wheelchair, she would wonder what had happened to that person, but she would not know how to respond. She now realised, for the most part, that people in wheelchairs were just like everyone else;

they had thoughts and feelings, memories and loved ones, worries, and dreams. They were people.

Michelle's feelings about her predicament were coming out. She wrote, by blinking, to her friends, "I am living in a body that doesn't work."

In talking to Michelle, Cori learned that Michelle was scared to go on the city bus because of the "other people." Michelle had never in the past cared about what others thought of her. But she was different now. In the past she had turned heads because of her beauty. Now people stared at her disabled, motionless body. She didn't want to go to the lobby of the hospital because other disabled residents wanted to talk to her, but she couldn't talk. It was heartbreaking for her to not be able to carry on a simple conversation. And the fact that merely holding up her head was something that she actually had "to think about all the time" only added to her frustration.

Cori was persistent in getting as much help for Michelle as possible. She was concerned about hand splints to keep Michelle's hands from curling. She wanted more information about Michelle's feeding tube. She thought there should be a reassessment of Michelle's swallowing abilities. She wanted to get Michelle swimming in the pool. Cori did get some action on her concerns. In regards to the splints, caregivers had contacted the orthotic specialist, and proper splints for Michelle's hands and feet were on order. The swimming pool was unfortunately temporarily closed, but her enrolment in a swimming program would be considered.

Mike recorded that Michelle had some active control in her left shoulder, chest muscle and biceps. Her right arm and hand continued to increase in function. But Michelle's head control was a totally different matter. It was noted that it would take a lot of re-training and strengthening before holding up her head would feel natural. Mike wrote, "We just have to keep working."

Another thing Cori was very concerned about was when Michelle had no call bell because her hand could not reach the switch. Cori wanted caregivers to come up with a solution for this problem as Michelle needed to be able to call for assistance whenever needed. Cori's fear for her sister was apparent when she wrote, "That must be scary!!!"

Michelle now had a daily routine very similar to what she had at Victoria General. Only the people were different. Tammi would continue to visit Michelle regularly, checking on her friend's condition, doing her nails, shaving her legs. She even noticed Michelle had a painful looking ingrown toenail that was infected and bleeding. She wanted to take care of it but was afraid of causing more harm. She would make sure someone looked into the situation.

It was noted that Michelle worked well with the EPSON, the machine that would help her communicate. It wasn't that Michelle did not have the intelligence to operate the EPSON. Her problem was with the slight movement of any part of her body, even her eyes. Her weak responses to commands to blink her eyes were slow and laborious, and often frustrating for everyone. For Michelle to say one word through the machine would take several minutes. An entire phrase or sentence would seem to take forever. Michelle was very aware that people would "talk over her." She was usually left out of the conversation. This bothered her.

Cori was frustrated with communication with the Epson. This was a tape machine that was like an accountant's adding machine, only it typed letters rather than numbers. Michelle would painstakingly enter messages into the machine during her alone time in the hospital. Cori remembered, "We would get one liners telling us what she did that day or what she wanted to wear the next day or what she would like us to get her from the store. I think it was frustrating for her to type much more than that to begin with. It was frustrating for us as family…because others would read them, then tear them off and put them places and ultimately those might be lost or thrown out and we couldn't get to read them and learn things from her. We used to write notes to everyone else to leave them alone and leave them on her machine so we, the family, could see them. Not much was private back then. Actually the lack of privacy bugged us all, but Michelle most of all."

Getting Michelle to move food quickly through her mouth was something therapists were working on. So far, she wasn't doing very well with this chore. But she was swallowing better, moving her Adam's apple upwards. She was given one eighth of a teaspoon of cranberry juice. She moved the juice slowly in her mouth, but had a slow swallowing response.

Nurses made a request for Cori to set up some phrases on the EPSON for Michelle to instruct the nurses on her needs for bathroom care. This way Michelle could let them know when she needed to relieve her bladder. Other phrases Michelle found useful were CU (can you please), DFW (don't feel well), HHA (have a headache), FG (feel good), and TSO (take splints off). These simple phrases helped Michelle deal with her daily needs without having to blink out the words at a snails pace on a letter board. It speeded things up.

Life in Michelle's new home carried on in a similar way to her stay in VGH, different people, different surroundings, but a familiar routine. But this was less of a hospital environment. It was important for caregivers at Gorge Road to help the residents return to normal social activities. And this was especially important to Michelle.

• • •

Sandy Fulton admitted that she was not really the right person to comment on Michelle's cognitive ability at that stage, however, she did have an interesting point of view. "I think she could figure things out but she couldn't express herself. I think intellectually she was intact. And there's a little bit of a difference between that (intellectual) and cognitive. Her brain was starved of oxygen, for sure, before she came into us. And, if she couldn't remember stuff, like somebody who was as bright as Michelle was, you would think she would remember, oh yeah, I was at GF Strong. And she's got a mind like a little steel trap, so why doesn't she remember. That's cognitive deficit. I think she could figure things out, and she absolutely knew when she was sad and she knew when she was happy and she knew that she hated it at the Gorge and she didn't want to be there. So, that's all kinds of thinking stuff, and cognition is thinking, right?"

Sandy offered some thoughts on Michelle's progress in Gorge Road. "From the Gorge they felt in January 2000 she (Michelle) was intellectually intact, had a sense of humour, challenged herself and was willing to try to learn. The fact that she couldn't is due to her brain injury, or to this injury which caused her brain injury. She's probably much more limited physically than she is intellectually. She's brighter on the inside than she is on the outside."

Chapter 22

It was January 7, 1994 and nineteen year old Michelle was embarking on a very adventurous vacation in Australia. She was sitting in the Auckland airport, preparing herself for a four hour wait. Time passed slowly as she wrote postcards and made a few phone calls. She was tired; one hour of sleep in the last 28 hours. It was a bit lonely, all on her own in a strange country. She was thinking she would definitely make sure she had at least one companion "next time."

The land in Australia, to Michelle, seemed very much like Victoria. The water was green and the hills were green, like Hawaii. Her flight had stopped in Fiji on route to Australia. Fiji was "very warm and muggy."

Don and Ella Nicolls were friends of the family and picked Michelle up from the airport. She wasn't to stay with the Nicolls for long, however, bush fires were burning all around Sydney and travelling was too dangerous. She wrote in her diary the first night in Sydney, "I was crazy to think of coming here by myself! But now I'm forcing myself to make the most of it and learn and grow from this situation I've put myself in!" Fortunately for Michelle, the Nicolls were "a great family."

On her first outing in Sydney, Michelle caught a ferry to Circular Quay and Darling Harbour. She visited the aquarium and noted in her diary she saw sharks, crocodiles, tropical fish and seals. "That was great!" She met a girl from Toronto and they went to a concert in Domain Park; listened to music, talked, and wrote some postcards. Then she took the ferry "home" where Don picked her up.

It was intriguing to Michelle how different the English language was in Australia. Words and phrases were completely new to her. She was learning new phrases such as "no worries" and "How hot is it?" which would mean to a Canadian "It's hot, eh?" The remark of "so stoked" implied the person was excited or thrilled. There were a few words that were quite different than the Canadian words. "Ice blocks" meant "ice cubes". "Cosie" meant "bathing suit." "Blarney" meant something like "darn."

The following day was a quiet, restful day. Michelle was dropped off at the beach where she spent a few hours. She did manage to get "a little color," however, the fires were creating a dense cloud of smoke and it was actually quite cold for a summer day.

After almost a week in Sydney, Michelle was ready to venture on. She hopped on a bus and travelled all night and all morning to Brisbane. There she waited for her next bus to Airlie Beach. It was another all night ride. When she arrived at Airlie and found the hostel, she "dumped my stuff in the room" and got herself organized. She planned her entire week in advance, booking buses and accommodation. It was now hot and sunny and she spent most of the day walking around, snacking on ice cream, or going for a swim when the heat was overwhelming. She loved it. "It's been a beautiful relaxing hot day! Just what I wanted!"

Michelle was already socializing. She met two other girls in her room. One, Sara, was from England and had been travelling for a year. The other girl, Susan, was American and was working in Korea. Michelle had fun that evening when she and Sara met up with some of Sara's friends at a local bar and grill. The meal was only four dollars and even included one drink. "That was great." The people she met were from all over the place. One guy was from Germany, and one from Colorado. There was a girl from Montreal and two other guys from Austria. "It was quite a group." They ate dinner, talked, played pool and danced. "It was great fun."

Michelle's only regret was that she hadn't booked more time to stay in Airlie. She really liked the place and decided she would have to go back again someday.

Her next excursion was to the Great Barrier Reef. "It took 2 hours to get there but it was worth it!" Michelle was fascinated by the coral and the fish. She took lots of pictures. The group snorkelled for about 2 hours then had a lunch. They sat around and suntanned for a while. Michelle covered herself with SPF-30 suntan lotion but still developed a slight burn.

On the trip back from the reef they stopped due to some boat trouble. While they waited, two dolphins came by. "It was wonderful." Back at the hostel Michelle spent a quiet evening, noting, "I can't move anyway."

The following day Michelle would be travelling again. Her bus did not leave until later on in the evening so she had many hours to kill. She was bored and found herself thinking about home and the situation there, her boyfriends, Wes and Jeff. But she was also enjoying her newfound freedom. "I have a feeling I'll have a big problem returning home where there's rules and parents and restrictions – how I act, where I am, what I'm doing, etc."

Michelle wrote some deep reflections in her diary about her boyfriends at home. She mentioned the great times she had experienced with Wes. They had been hanging out together for over three years. But there were good and there were bad times. She felt bad about the way she treated Wes, "other guys, drinking." And she was sorry she had hurt him. She was now comfortable with her decision that the two of them be friends only, "although I'll always love him dearly."

Then there was Jeff. He gave her butterflies. She was excited and nervous about seeing him when she got back home. She was afraid of "screwing up." She didn't want to be hurt, and she didn't want to hurt him. Yet she knew they could have some good times together and lots of fun. "I want to take it as it comes."

She caught her bus that evening and travelled all night, arriving in Hervey Bay at 9 in the morning. "Boy, was I tired!" A fellow named Jimmy picked her up with his red jeep and took her to Olympus, a brand new backpacker's villa. It was a beautiful place, about 10 minutes from the beach. The unit had a kitchen and common room which had a TV and a bathroom and more beds. Upstairs was a toilet and shower, more beds and another lounging area. There was also a deck that overlooked the pool. Michelle thought it was great.

She met lots of people. One girl was from Toronto and two others were from Ottawa. There was a guy from Israel and a girl from Austria, a couple from Germany and two fellows from Sydney. Michelle had a long interesting talk about travelling with Jay, a young guy from Germany. There was lots of time for visiting. The weather was terrible. It was cloudy and dull, and a full cyclone warning for Brisbane to Mackay. It rained all afternoon. This was a good day to visit with other interesting travellers.

Michelle was amazed with what she was discovering about herself in her free time. She had decided she was really interested in getting into the field of Resort Management and maybe even getting a business degree to go with it. She felt she was ready to work harder. She wanted to "work-out and get healthy." She also thought she could work two jobs and get two years of "top grades." Her final goal told of her strong desire for independence when she wrote, "And hopefully move out!"

Michelle's next stop was Byron Bay. It was raining and miserable. But the hostel was fantastic. It was set up like a hotel, the rooms encircling a pool. The weather cleared the following day and Michelle joined a guy, Tim, on a trail up to a lighthouse. From the view up there of the ocean they saw a sting ray and dozens of dolphins. There were also some goats around the lighthouse. It was fun.

They went to the beach for some sun tanning and swimming. Michelle, with her fair skin, took in a little too much sun. Again. She partied that evening until quite late. There was wine. Everyone finally called it a night, except for Michelle and Tim. They had this crazy idea of swimming in the ocean at one in the morning. In the dark, fully clothed, half drunk, they both went running into the water. Michelle wrote later in her diary, "It was rather fun."

Michelle took the bus back to Sydney and, once again, stayed with the Nicolls. Now that she was back living with the adults, she was missing home and her fellow peers. "I miss Cori and Jeff a lot!"

The following day Michelle visited the zoo and saw koalas, kangaroos and platypus. She thought the koalas were "absolutely adorable." Her new friend, Tim, was supposed to meet her there, but they somehow missed each other. She was later than expected and figured he had simply tired of waiting. She found out later that he had been there about the same time but they must have passed each other in the water. She was very upset about it "especially when I was looking forward to the company so much." Michelle found herself starving for "people interaction."

Her next adventure was sightseeing at Wynyard. She hung around the harbour, fascinated by the street workers. She amused herself watching the acts and listening to music. All sorts of goods were for sale: pottery, jewellery, rocks, gems, hats and lots of art. She wandered down to the Opera House, checked it out, and finally made her way back to Newport where Don picked her up. Michelle had a final dinner with the Nicolls. She was to fly to New Zealand in the morning. She felt they had been so nice to her and she made a note to send them a huge thank you note.

New Zealand reminded Michelle of Canada's Rocky Mountains. It was lush and green. The temperature was more moderate, cooler than Australia. She stayed at Elm Lodge in Dunedin.

This is where she spent her first day, checking out the town. There were lots of things to see, the Art Centre, Botanical Gardens, the Museum, and Cathedral Square. She even went to church. She finished off the day with some shopping. Back at her room she planned her route for the next day and packed up.

In the morning she got out of bed early and caught a bus that took her to a train. This took her to another hostel. She booked a tour of Otego Peninsula and was quite fascinated with her visit to a sheep farm and an albatross colony. She saw fur seals and penguins. She was stunned at how close she could walk to the seals, almost stumbling over them as the round creatures blended into the rocks. She learned that Blue penguins were the smallest penguins in the world and, when they shed their feathers, it was called "fluffing." The tour group also hiked through a sheep and cow field to get to the area of the sea lions. Michelle loved the hike. The sea lions, she noted, were much larger than the seals and more aggressive. The group of people were chased by a couple of them. She had a great time.

Michelle caught a bus to Queenstown the following day and arrived just in time to get onto the Dart River Jet Boat Safari. She and a few others were taken on a speedy ride up the river; the driver thrilled them with quick turns and 360s. Along the way, they were shown some beautiful waterfalls. It was on this ride that Michelle met two Melbourne fellows, Jason and Andrew.

The two guys asked Michelle if she would like to travel with them to Milford Sound and she decided to live a little and go along. "Well, it was quite the adventure just getting there. We were dodging possums and rabbits along the road and unfortunately we hit a rabbit I think, and we definitely mutilated a possum. I was so grossed out!" But the view of the night sky and the mountains was gorgeous. Michelle wound up roughing it a little more than expected. The hostel in the area was closed and she had not brought along with her a sleeping bag or mat. The men pitched a tent and loaned her a couple of sweaters to keep her warm. Andrew let her use the lining of his sleeping bag and Jason let her use his mat. She slept in between them.

The three travellers spent some time discovering Milford Sound, taking some pictures. They moved on to Mount Cook where they rode a gondola to the top and took in a spectacular view. They watched the bungy jumpers and the soft parachute parapenters for a while, and returned to the bottom of the mountain for a KFC dinner. Michelle's mother did not seem happy when she learned in a phone call that Michelle was travelling with two men. Michelle wrote in her diary about this. "But there's no worries here. These guys are great (they'll even open doors for me)."

It was a good thing Michelle's mom did not know of the antics that went on that evening. Michelle, Andrew and Jason decided at 12 am to go for a walk. They sat on the road, talking and looking at the stars. They returned to the hostel around 2 am and "the fun began, pillow stealing, pillow fights, tickling! I think we finally got to sleep (all in one room, Jason was on the floor between beds) around 6 am. And we were up at 9 am." And the evening after that Michelle went to dinner at an Irish bar with her two male companions along with another two of their friends. She and the four guys had such a good time. Michelle laughed so hard over their "sick sense of humour."

It was five days, the best of days. Michelle had a wonderful time with Jason and Andrew. They ate, they drank, they talked and laughed, they partied. She felt sick having to say goodbye to them. They all parted with promises to keep in touch.

Michelle was spending a couple of days at a "hippy place!" The fellow running it was "really laid back." The peace and quiet allowed Michelle to think of her return to Canada. In less than a month, she would be going home, and she was making plans. "I want to buy a bike, join the gym full blast and get my mind set to study hard for 2 years. I'm definitely doing two jobs when I get home. The busier the better! No more TV either! No more junk, no more indecision, no more self-pity, no more alcohol! I've never had such a clear view of this before. I get up, walk/exercise, bike to work, bike home, dinner, gym, homework, friends. I really want – need – to be healthy and feeling good."

Michelle's travels had changed her way of thinking of herself. She felt alive, "indestructible." To her "Down Under" was very organic. She felt that the way she conducted her life in Canada left her "stale." She realized that back in Canada she was not doing enough to be healthy.

Michelle's thoughts on her future were totally different now. She spoke to her parents on the phone who mentioned to her how stressed one of Michelle's friends was about school. Michelle laughed out loud. She knew she would never again allow stress to control her life. Now she would "think of Jason, Andrew, Katie, Dave and Marcus! And Doug and Andy! I've decided that if Jason and Andrew haven't come to Canada in two years, I'm going to Australia to find them and maybe work in a hotel or backpackers…my life is going to be exciting from now on! No more half living! I want to live each day to the fullest…meaning skydiving this summer, Kim's wedding …biking every day, going to the gym, seeing Jeff and having fun…Also horseback riding and waterskiing, tubing, parasailing."

One of Michelle's most exciting adventures in Australia was skydiving. "9000 feet and we jumped 5000 free fall and then floated 4000! Unreal! I can't even describe the feeling but I'll never forget it!"

Travelling on to New Zealand, Michelle's vacation involved sightseeing, boat riding, swimming and sun tanning. She called her mother and asked her to book a doctor appointment for her. Her mom asked if she was pregnant. This comment made Michelle go to the doctor right away. The test was negative. Michelle's boyfriend at home, Jeff, had been worried. This would be good news for him.

Then she met up with a gang of people her age and the partying began. There was lots of beer, lots of laughs and many late nights. Michelle had some late night chats with a few of the guys she'd met. One fellow mentioned that she would go far in her life, that she was confident of herself. She replied that her confidence was only on the outside.

The end of Michelle's vacation was creeping closer. She flew to Fiji and spent her first night in a beautiful room with two full beds. She had it all to herself, which was a wonderful change. She met a nice group of travellers here. They enjoyed some sightseeing and, of course, some night life, which also included some drinking. Some of them tried snorkelling and scuba diving and a few of them attempted some of the local dance moves. Michelle very much enjoyed the dancing.

Michelle discovered while talking to her companions that one guy was a doctor and another was an engineer. This fascinated her, that they were so "on the ball."

On her second last night in Fiji Michelle partied most of the evening and woke up the next day feeling terrible. She spent most of the day resting in the shade. She went on a beautiful sunset cruise for her last evening in Fiji. "It was pure heaven."

On her flight back to Canada, Michelle wrote, "And so my trip is coming to an end after an 18 hour plane ride. Sad really! I had a good time!

• • •

Jason Clappison was a young fellow from Australia who was travelling with a "mate". They were visiting Christchurch, New Zealand, wasting a couple of days before picking up their "push bikes" from the port and beginning an 1800 kilometer trek around the south island. Jason, with his dark, almost shoulder length hair enjoyed cycling and was in solid physical condition. The two men had decided to stay along their way at hostels. This way it would be more affordable for them, and they would also meet other travelers who were normally interested in meeting people and having a good time. According to Jason, "We got that right."

Jason was staying at a hostel called Foley Towers. It was run by a Canadian. Jason called him an American and was "rightly chastised." Jason was in the living room of the hostel when he saw Michelle sitting in the corner reading a book. He had always been attracted to girls who looked after themselves and took good care of their appearance. Michelle was definitely one of those girls. In Jason's eyes, "She didn't have to work too hard at it. She has a natural beauty and attraction about her that her bright blue eyes set alight." When Michelle laughed it seemed to be reflected in those eyes and he could tell her laughter was purely genuine.

To Jason, Michelle did not "create a veil or an emotional barrier" that he had seen in a lot of other people. He was impressed by Michelle's independent action of travelling on her own. With Jason it would normally take him a long time to allow himself to get close to someone, but it was easy for him to connect with Michelle. She was very considerate and easy to get along with. They simply enjoyed each other's company, doing things together like sight-seeing, breakfast, lunch and dinner, and shopping.

When they finally had to say goodbye and return to their own far away homes, it was very emotional for Jason. He did not want her to leave, and yet he knew they would see each other again. And they never really lost contact over the years. Jason had in his mind to someday travel to Canada and visit Michelle.

Jason read about Michelle's "tragic event" in an email. It was difficult for him to believe such a terrible thing could happen to such a special person. He felt that "if I could do anything to change it, I would."

Jason found within his own life that he would use Michelle's situation as an example and a motivation "to live life like today is your last." He realized that his attitude sounded rather final, "but her independence had been stolen and I'm not sure how I would handle such a thing."

• • •

There is an Australian expression, "fair dinkum", which would be like a Canadian saying "OK, whatever." This was how Jason came across to Michelle. Even though Jason was generally a serious person, Michelle enjoyed his good sense of humour and his relaxed disposition. Their friendship has endured.

Chapter 23

Michelle was taken to the hospital for a small operation. The tube going into her stomach had to be changed. When brought back to Gorge Road, Michelle informed her sister that she had been awake all through the surgery and had felt everything. It hurt. And she cried. Thankfully she was put on morphine shortly after the procedure was completed. This was something Michelle would experience from time to time. It was actually not a surgery but a simple task of removing the gastric tube from her stomach. The tube was replaced with a new one that was held in place by a small balloon that would be inflated inside the stomach.

Cori was very excited when, a few days later, Michelle initiated a conversation for the very first time. Cori noted that Michelle changed the subject, asked questions, and purposefully continued the conversation. Cori could tell that this also excited Michelle. It was a turning point in Michelle's recovery.

Michelle had now progressed to moving her right hand and arm quite well. She could bend her elbow from straight out, back to her waist, and return it out again. She was also trying very hard to talk. Some people mentioned that she would try to say "thank you." Tammi said, "She'll be talking in no time."

The days passed. Once in a while it was noted that Michelle had a bad day. One day she had all of her hair cut off. A new style for her? She received a new Kincontrol box, remote control and all. This would be of great benefit to her. Tammi would still do her nails periodically. One day she did them in white with red hearts.

Everyone was trying to take care of Michelle. Cori asked for help in pumping up the wheels of Michelle's chair. Her armrest had also fallen off and Cori needed help in putting it back on. Mike, the OT, was hounding Cori to spend some time with him to learn certain therapies to give to Michelle. Cori was working and had exams to mark. Sometimes it was all so overwhelming.

Cori arrived at Gorge Road one day to find Michelle crying. Michelle indicated that "it is not fair for you." Cori told her sister that it was fine and she wouldn't change a thing. Michelle's sense of compassion for her sister's struggle was monumental. It was a good indication of Michelle's characteristic concern for others. Michelle worried about being a burden to her family. She hated not being able to look after herself.

Shopping was a unique experience now. Michelle would be gawked at or, most often, entirely ignored. However, once in a while she would meet a person who had the uncanny sense of knowing how to deal with her, somebody who would have the patience to wait for Michelle's slow communication. One clerk remarked, "What a neat sign language with your eyes!" Some people looked at her as a real person. It was remarkable.

From time to time Michelle was taken via HandyDART to join a family gathering. They all seemed to embrace the way things were now. The family usually had a good time, and Michelle, in her wheelchair, was frequently included. Although her communication was painfully slow, she could understand and join in the conversation, albeit in a small way.

Michelle wanted more therapy done with her mouth. She could now take small sips of thickened liquid. But her problem was controlling it with her mouth. Her lips and tongue were extremely weak. When it came to Michelle's Epson communicating device, she was doing a great job, making "long sentences, faster, accurate."

Things were beginning to happen in Michelle's life. There were plans to take her to the movies. There were plans to take her to the pub. Tammi and another friend, Chris, took Michelle to downtown Victoria where they visited the London Wax Museum and Miniature World. "We were all tired!!"

Michelle's life was more active during her stay at the Gorge Road facility. There was a hotel right next door, which included a pub and a night club. Care aids would take a group of residents to the pub from time to time, and occasionally some would stay later to take in the night club. Michelle would enjoy these excursions, feeling once again a sense of normalcy.

Michelle maintained a positive attitude. She was easy-going and helpful with the nurses. She worked hard in her physiotherapy, improving the strength in the fingers of her right hand, and beginning to move her shoulder. She could hold her head up by herself for long periods of time and was trying her best to swallow. Physiotherapy was very important to her. She wanted to get better. And she would become very upset if there was a lack of attention in this regard.

Physiotherapy involved many things. Her limbs would be stretched and she would be helped through resistance exercises. Mike would even challenge her to some arm wrestling. Gorge Road also had a pool, so she also did some exercise in the water. This way she could actually stand, although with a lot of help. It was hard work for the therapists to hold her upright. Teresa, another of her therapists, gave muscle stimulation to her right arm. With the current of a couple of electrodes taped over a certain muscle, Michelle practiced lifting a Beanie Baby. Teresa was a great helper with Michelle. She was fun, maybe a little sarcastic, but that's what Michelle thought was funny. It was the differing personalities of her therapists and caregivers that provided Michelle with some degree of entertainment.

The Epson communicator became a lifeline for Michelle. Sometimes it would go "haywire" and Michelle would be left with very little means to join in a conversation. Or visitors would come in to find a visibly upset and anxious Michelle with her control frustratingly out of reach.

Michelle went to her first concert since her stroke. The artist, Julian Austin, kissed Michelle and gave her a hug, promising to have front row tickets for her for his next concert. It was so wonderful that friends and family appreciated Michelle's need for a social, active life. They did their very best, despite all the difficulties, to provide this for her. Michelle recalls what a good time she had at the concert, and that "being in a wheelchair is sometimes really a bonus, people feel sorry for you." She knew there was no way she would have ever met Julian otherwise.

Karen, Michelle's speech therapist, mentioned that she tried to give Michelle a dab of apple sauce. Unfortunately, Michelle still had difficulty moving solids around with her tongue. Karen would continue to try to give Michelle small tastes of juice. Karen also reminded everyone that it was important for all to remember to charge Michelle's Epson for the next day's use. Otherwise Michelle would not be able to communicate.

A splint was fitted for Michelle's left foot. This would help lengthen the Achilles tendon and help prevent foot drop. This was something that her dad had fought for. It was a constant battle for him. He tried very hard to make certain Michelle had the very best of care.

Eventually Michelle began "serial casting" where she first had "bivalve casts". Her feet were casted into the correct position. The casts were cut along each side so they could be removed when need be. To keep the casts on, they were wrapped with a tenser bandage. The casts would be regularly removed so that Michelle's feet could be examined for pressure sores.

Michelle also endured Botox injections into her calf muscles. The purpose of the injections was to help relax the muscles and hopefully prevent spasms and tightening. Also, it was imperative to Michelle to keep herself in the very best physical condition possible. She would say, "Why go through this torture? And, yes, it is torture, but I am convinced that there will be a breakthrough soon and I should be in good shape. Also it's easier to put shoes on if they're straighter."

• • •

GF Strong Rehabilitation Centre was the place Michelle wanted to be. She knew she would receive the best therapy there. Her mother joined Michelle on an excursion by ferry to Vancouver to GF Strong where Michelle was to meet the staff. It was a long trip for Michelle, having to hold up her head for such a lengthy time. Her neck was very sore. When they arrived at GF Strong, staff immediately took care of her, getting her settled and working on her painful neck.

The plan was for Michelle to learn Morse code so that she could operate a more sophisticated Epson machine and, eventually, have her own computer. A bonus for Michelle being at GF Strong was that staff would take her for therapy three times a day. They were also trying to work with her on using a bedpan and it seemed to be successful most of the time. Michelle was booked for a Barium swallow test to check out her ability in this area.

• • •

There was another wonderful turn of events for Michelle. A good family friend had decided that the community "should get behind Michelle and help her with her plight." This family friend discussed with Joan and Gordon how the family might feel about a community project. He wanted to know if they would welcome this plan, or would they be embarrassed? Gordon was a well-known person in the community and a public school administrator. As Gordon put it, "My professional position was sound and my income was not low, nor in any jeopardy." They were also concerned as to how Michelle would feel being a "public" figure, noted in the news, and being publicly featured with her disability.

When it was decided to go ahead with the fundraiser, it was clear that the family's involvement with music and the church and the community would dictate the direction of the funding plan. Gordon had spent a good deal of time with local choirs where all three of his children had participated from time to time. Gordon's friend came up with the idea of using the Sagebrush (community) Theatre for an evening of choral music, featuring choirs from around Kamloops. As the planning of the event progressed, eight choirs offered to participate. The audience was to purchase tickets for the choral evening, and choir members not only sang but also paid for a ticket themselves to add to the donations. Publicity of the entertainment happened through word of mouth in the community, along with mention on the radio and articles in the newspaper.

A flyer was made that explained Michelle's situation. It read like this: *Michelle Britton – Michelle was born in Kamloops on May 28, 1974, to Gordon & Joan Britton. She led a very full and exciting life, including music, dancing, downhill, water and cross country skiing, swimming and hiking, etc. She was happy and popular wherever she went. Michelle was Co-Valedictorian of her graduating class in Grade 12 from Westsyde Senior Secondary School. She went to UCC and received her two year diploma in Hotel Management. This took her to the Rimrock Hotel in Banff for five months for her concluding practicum. Travel then took her to Australia and New Zealand for some months. On return she decided to take advantage of the University of Victoria's program by which her two year Diploma would be accepted as the first two years of a four year Bachelor's Degree in Commerce. Michelle had just completed this degree in the spring of 1999 except for the attached work experience.*

The event of May 17, 1999 was to change her life forever. Walking across the lawn at UVic. Michelle collapsed and was rushed to Hospital. After two days in ICU it was determined that she had suffered a Spontaneous Arterial Dissection, in effect, a stroke, and was paralyzed from the mouth down. There was no prognosis. It was a wait and see game plan, with blood thinners, other medications, some measure of life support, and care. Quite soon thereafter, feeling returned to her body, and some indication of muscle tone became apparent. Communication was established with eye blink for "yes" and "no". After two months the tracheotomy tube was removed and she could begin to feel "normal" around her face. An intravenous tube remained for medications. Since that time, that tube has been removed and she has only the "peg" for feeding directly into her stomach. Over the last few months, family, friends and hospital staff have provided care, treatment, and encouragement. The result is some progress. Michelle has muscular tone in her neck, mouth area, right forearm, fingers, leg, foot, and to some extent, toes. She has continued to keep a cheerful attitude and is determined to beat this affliction. Michelle works at improving all the time, to the extent that she can.

Many of us are determined to do all we can to further therapy and see the continued improvements to her condition. Where this will end, we do not know. We are insistent on finding all the help, as long as it takes, to get her to as much "normal" life as possible.

Our goal was to get Michelle to the GF Strong centre in Vancouver. We were convinced that this was the best hope for her continued recovery. A three week assessment at GF Strong grew to a seven-week session during which she learned Morse code to communicate through a finger operated switch into an Epson communication board. It was also determined what physical therapy would be most useful to her development, and the form of controls needed for her to operate a motorized wheelchair. In addition a start was made to oral feeding.

Currently, Michelle resides in an extended care section of Gorge Road Hospital in Victoria. Other more appropriate residences are being considered and one day Michelle may well move to a residence more suitable for her age and capabilities. The goal is to achieve as much independent living as possible.

Some of the many additional items Michelle will be needing are listed below:

Physiotherapist @ $55.00 per week
Hydraulic Lift @ $3,000.00
Wheelchair-accessible Van @ $50,000.00
Motorized Bed @ $3,000.00

Computerized Communication System @ $15,000.00
Independent Living Support @ $3,000.00 per month
Misc. Medical Support Equipment @ $6,000.00

Hopefully you and all her many other friends will see fit to help her along the way.

It was a huge success! The theatre was jammed. The attending audience was thrilled with the program and very touched when Michelle and her family were introduced on stage. And what followed was truly amazing. Not only did the event generate a decent collection of funds, but a bank account was created for further donation towards Michelle's needs. This bank account grew amazingly to about $50,000. This, of course, would lead to a new problem for the family. What would they do with the money? How could they best serve Michelle's needs with the astounding generosity of their community friends? A decision was made to purchase a wheelchair accessible van, and a search began. Eventually, a 1997 Dodge Grand Caravan, currently in use at that time, was found in Ladner. A member of Michelle's uncle's church, a wheelchair bound man himself, had a surplus van to his rental fleet, and agreed to sell it. After an inspection by BCAA, and an agreement made on the price, the van was purchased.

The van was "a great blessing to Michelle, enabling such mobility." Gordon mentioned how they owed so much to the friend who initially came up with the fundraising idea and took it upon himself to organize the entire project and see it through to completion. "Such a blessing!"

• • •

On a sunny April day Cori and Michelle travelled to the Westwood Plateau Golf Club. It was here that their cousin, Kathy, was married. Wedding planners made sure Michelle was seated where she could see everything. They watched Kathy walk down the aisle to a swing/

jive song. They were "in awe of her." They stayed for the buffet dinner and a few speeches. It was a beautiful wedding. But it was difficult for Michelle. The happiness of the bride and groom made it so obvious to Michelle what she was missing in her own life. She could not control her inner sadness.

On May 28 Michelle celebrated her twenty sixth birthday. She and Cori travelled on the HandyDART to the Seabus where they went from the North Shore to West Vancouver. This was where her grandparents threw her a birthday party. There were cards, gifts, friends and family. And ice cream cake. It was not the kind of celebration Michelle expected she would be having at the age of 26. She and her friends would probably have gone to a pub or two and partied all night long, drinking, and dancing and doing all the crazy things young people do. Now she was in a wheelchair, her partying days over. She always loved her grandparents' house in West Vancouver. She was happy to be there. But she felt "stuck." She couldn't just go check out the upstairs, or go down to the basement. How would she ever deal with this new life?

• • •

Cori wrote in her own diary about her boyfriend, Javier: "It's an amazing feeling. And the whole family loves him. They really do! I'm elated about it all. Yet, it's been a hard year since Michelle's "accident". And I'm still dealing with it. Really dealing with it. I have huge guilt trips and then swings of sadness and then, sense of loss, all mixed in with joys of seeing Michelle and loving the times spent with her and feelings of such closeness!! All at once, sometimes, which is too difficult to handle. And at those times, I really, really appreciate having Javier around to help me through it. If he's not near, the family is but it's not the same. I really miss the old times with my sister. But, I'm glad I met Javier."

However, the relationship between Cori and Javier was strained. Cori wrote Javier a letter: "…how much I care for you and love you and want you in my life. But I also feel so much else.

"I feel loss and grief for the sister that I once had. And this is the biggest thing I've ever had to deal with. It's hard to handle. I've 'lost' my best friend.

"I feel anger that it had to happen to her and not someone else. I feel anger that my parents aren't here more. I feel anger that I've found you during the worse period of my life and I can't really enjoy it because of all the other things. I feel anger. Lots and lots. AND I'm SO SORRY I TAKE IT OUT ON YOU. I'M SORRY.

"I feel quite empty of happiness right now. Please don't take that personally. It has nothing to do with you. You are my sanctuary and the person with whom I can relax (even if you don't believe that). I think of you when I'm most depressed or upset and I feel better. It's true.

"I can't handle any changes right now. That is, I am very stressed if something in my plan for the day is changed. If you remember all of the times I have been stressed will be times that my plan was different. I can't adapt so quickly anymore. I need a safe environment that won't rock me or push me off my balance. In this safe place, I can handle my life. You are part of my safe place."

• • •

A great milestone was achieved. Michelle drove a power wheelchair for the first time. She operated the machine with a touch pad that was controlled with her right fingers. She drove on her own around the gym for more than two hours. This was a huge sense of freedom and independence.

Michelle's eyes were tested to evaluate her vision for reading. It was discovered that her right eye had double vision. An eye-patch over this eye would hopefully help.

Back at Gorge Road, Cori wrote an update on everything that had been happening in Michelle's life. Cori and her parents were working on finding a private home for Michelle, perhaps in Kamloops. They were also trying to find her a motorized wheelchair. Their goal was to do all they could to provide Michelle with a better quality life.

Michelle's communicating device, the Epson, was the very most important tool she could have. This machine helped her voice her opinions, her needs, and her wants for her future. It was imperative that the machine be charged overnight and set up for Michelle each morning. It would not be long, however, until Michelle would receive her very own computer which would change her life in enormous ways when it came to conversing with others. She would now be able to talk, albeit still awfully slowly. But she would be able to form complete sentences conveying her own personal ideas in regards to her daily life and her future, using her computer and Morse code.

An update was needed on Michelle's medications. The Zoloft, which was to improve her mood, was to be decreased to the point where she would hopefully not need it at all. However, nobody seemed to know the process of doing this. Michelle never thought she needed Zoloft and she wanted to be off it completely. Coumadin, a blood thinner, was another drug Michelle was taking. And it was thought that she no longer needed this drug. There was a question on this. Michelle also took a continual medication to help her bowels move properly.

Cori wrote a list of physiotherapies for Michelle. Mike and Deb were to take Michelle upstairs for one hour of therapy each day. Mike was to later give Michelle 35 minutes more work. Massage therapists in training volunteered to work with Michelle as often as possible. And Cori herself was to exercise Michelle's arms and legs two times a week.

When it came to eating and speaking there was more and more improvement. Michelle was eating yogurt and pudding. The muscles of her throat and mouth were strengthening. She made sounds and moved her lips to try and shape words.

Notes were written quite often in Michelle's diary about her equipment. It was an ongoing effort to keep all of the gadgets working properly. Her Kincontrol, which operated the radio and call bell had to be programmed so that one specific number operated the radio and another the call bell. For people who were not specially trained with these machines, it could be a challenging task keeping everything in working order. Cori tried to keep on top of it, but even she often needed the help of a technical expert. Occasionally it would be noted that the Epson had not been charged the night before. This would be a constant frustration for Michelle.

Patsy, a volunteer, spent time with Michelle and would take her on outings. They went to the mall and Patsy helped Michelle buy a top and some birthday cards. She would take Michelle outside for a walk and would read to her. Michelle wanted to venture down certain pathways, but Patsy was cautious not to take Michelle into any areas that may put her in jeopardy. There were also days when Michelle was simply not up to a venture and was sometimes letting her emotions get the best of her. Michelle thought Patsy was a "really nice lady". She was a petite blonde. "Lots of fun." Michelle felt Patsy really cared about her well-being. She didn't take "crap" from people and was very protective of Michelle. Patsy knew that Michelle was quite conscious of people staring at her. Patsy would tell Michelle to ignore it.

Someone had filed an application to the provincial Ministry for financial assistance in purchasing Michelle a power wheelchair. As expected, it was denied. The social worker would file an appeal on behalf of Michelle. This was the typical "red tape" that Michelle and those around her became accustomed to when dealing with the government. Everything was challenging and totally exasperating.

It was a few months later that Michelle received her new power wheelchair. This would be a turning point in her life. Even the occupational therapist, Allison, was delighted. She wrote: "New Power Chair Arrives! Michelle was set up today in the power wheelchair. She took to it like a duck to water! She's still getting the hang of using the finger touch pod but she's doing great so far."

On a day close to Christmas, Patsy wrote: "Michelle and I spent time together, read, tidied room. She gave me a gift for which I have never been more touched in all my life. She has taught me more about strength and the human spirit than I will ever know. I don't often meet angels, but I have met one. Merry Christmas."

On December 19, 2000, Michelle travelled by HandyDART to the ferry at Swartz Bay that took them over the water to Tsawwassen. Then they drove to Kamloops in her new van. Gordon had fixed up the place in preparation for Michelle's stay. He had built a wheelchair ramp for access to the back entrance. In the ceiling of her old bedroom a lift system had been installed for Michelle to assist her into bed. Three student nurses were there at the house to help Michelle settle into her room. She was home.

• • •

In September, 2000, Dr. R. LaFreniere wrote this consultation report:

This 26-year-old lady was seen in the GRH extended care unit on the 18th of September, 2000.

She is an unfortunate young lady, who has had massive damage to the pons and cerebellum following what appears to have been a vertebral artery dissection occurring on the 17th of May, 1999. She was found in the UVIC parking lot and was brought into hospital. Investigations were done and the end result was someone with essentially a locked-in syndrome. She was transferred to GRH extended care where she has been since 30th of November, 1999.

In May of this year, she went to GF Strong to further look at her communication abilities and has since returned.

Her examination shows her to have fairly limited abilities to move. According to her physiotherapist, she is able to do a little bit of movement about the scapula, has slight bit of triceps, but none of this is very functional. She does have some right wrist extension, a bit of flexion, a bit of pronation, supination. She also has intermittently some biceps, though I didn't see this today. She is able to move her fingers, though not necessarily all independently and not with great control. She also, has, according to the therapist, a little bit of non-functional movement in the right leg, but nothing essentially on the left. She can turn her head independently. She can blink for communication and this seems to be somewhat effective.

Her augmented communication has been with an Epson machine, which is admittedly a bit dated, but through which she communicates with Morse code, ending up with a printed output. I have spoken to the OT who is also working with speech therapy, and who will try to further refine the system that they have currently. The plans are to move initially to a Macintosh system and eventually onto a lap top with voice synthesis, though that is still some ways down the road.

From the point of view of motor return, she has essentially reached a plateau quite some time ago and the therapist says that he has not seen any changes in her since she has gone to GF Strong and perhaps even somewhat before that. I would therefore be somewhat pessimistic with regards to further motor return at this point.

It would appear that the direction is towards a better system and I think that the OT has a pretty good grasp of what will work and what will be required.

• • •

A report was written on a Modified Barium Swallow test for Michelle:

The patient was given initially a thick mixture. This demonstrated very slow oral transit with gradual spillage over the back of the tongue and pooling of the valleculae and piriform sinuses. With gradual filling of the valleculae, this triggered a swallow. The larger bolus actually triggered a quicker swallow. A semi-thick mixture demonstrated a similar pattern of swallowing. There was good laryngeal elevation. There was however a tiny trace of aspiration. Pudding mixture demonstrated similar pattern with a minimal trace of aspiration. A thin mixture demonstrated a reduced swallowing reflex.

Chapter 24

Gorge Road Hospital was Michelle's home for two years. During this time her physical abilities continued to improve, but gains were nominal, and it became clear to most of those in the healthcare industry that Michelle's life would be forever considerably limited.

GF Strong was British Columbia's state of the art rehabilitation centre. Those who had experienced strokes or spinal cord injuries were benefited greatly by receiving daily therapy at this wonderful place. However, if there was little improvement in a person's condition within the first few months following the injury, it was unlikely that a regiment of therapy at GF Strong would be of any help.

Unfortunately for Michelle, her assessment at GF Strong determined that her ability to move the majority of her body was highly compromised. Michelle was substantially disabled, and it was thought that no amount of therapy would make a significant difference to her daily abilities.

Therefore, her application to receive extensive therapy at GF Strong was denied.

Michelle and her family were now on their own, taking on the huge responsibility of improving her life. It was a daily struggle that would turn into weeks, months, and years.

• • •

Cori reminisced in her diary: "I was thinking earlier about Michelle's past and how different it is/was to now. I was staring at her computer print-out of her standing along the ocean (?) in the wind in Nova Scotia (taken April 1999), just one month before her "accident." Looking at that picture made me think of her wild times and all her travelling. And flying, etc. She always seemed to enjoy life, and do as she liked regardless of everyone. (Happy face inserted here) And you know, it's a very good thing she did. How we would all kick ourselves if we had stopped or grounded her. (Just try it, eh?) (Happy face drawn here) But, it is almost like Michelle knew something was going to stop her from continuing her activities. Something driving her to experience a lot before she can't any longer."

• • •

The first plan for Michelle was put into motion by a large number of people in the healthcare industry. There were meetings between various professionals involved in Michelle's care. There were the doctors and nurses and District Health personnel. Angel Medical Equipment Supplier, which took care of such needs as wheelchairs, lifts, lift motors, ceiling brackets and tracking, was included in discussions. Other important people to Michelle's care were the occupational therapy personnel, CSIL program personnel, the Vancouver Island Health Authority, and Human Resources. There was also the nutritionist, the speech pathologist and an agency entitled TIL, (Technology in Living), that supported people with disability needs. All of these people got together and consulted over Michelle's physical placement outside of Gorge Road Hospital.

Copies of Michelle's medical records showed 29 handwritten pages documenting the incredibly complicated process of planning to move Michelle out of the system and back into society.

Joan and Gordon were amazed at the time that was given to organize Michelle's move. Gordon would say, "It was a cast of thousands." The entire process was complicated and fairly lengthy. Gordon could remember times when there were ten or twelve people sitting around a table "discussing the ramifications of the move." Although Michelle and her family were consulted throughout the process, in actuality, they were merely observers of a complex endeavour of the professionals. Luckily, those tireless people were in total control of searching out locations, making decisions on logistics, and providing much needed finances.

Subsidized housing was always in short supply in Victoria. As caregiver personnel explored the possibilities, a townhouse in a complex called "Jolly Place" became available. Michelle's new home was provided by an organization called Pacifica Housing Society. New residents were required to meet the criteria of being disabled and have low income, along with other specific needs.

The CSIL (Choice in Supports for Independent Living) required Joan and Gordon to register as a Society on behalf of Michelle in order to manage Michelle's CSIL program funding, which would finance the wages of caregivers. It was Joan's and Gordon's responsibility to search out the helpers for Michelle. It was also their task to provide furniture for the townhouse. Another job for them was to create guidelines and procedures for caregivers to follow when exercising Michelle's daily care.

Fortunately, Joan and Gordon did not have to deal with the Ministry. Michelle was under the responsibility of Vancouver Island Health Authority (VIHA). She was classified as Disability II and qualified for the maximum support. Financial assistance of $6000.00 per month was provided for her daily care and living expenses. This would include paying for caregiver help 24 hours a day, 7 days a week. The money would also assist in normal living costs such as utilities and food.

Finding homecare staff for Michelle was not easy. Joan and Gordon (the Society) now had the duty of seeking out suitable staff through newspaper advertisements. They trained and supervised this person once they were hired, and provided a pay cheque. This new "job" for the aging Britton parents was often a nightmare of dealing with an array of problems they would never have expected to come their way at this point in the lives. Who would have thought they would be burdened with the chore of providing complete care for a 26-year-old child/woman who, in the normal progression of life, should have been heading towards a career job, marriage and children. Joan and Gordon questioned their own future; their retirement. They had been only months away from achieving the "down-time" that all hard working people aspire to when entering their "golden" years. They were ready to do some major travelling. Everything they had worked for and dreamt of would now include a coating of guilt.

When the townhouse at Jolly Place became available, Michelle needed a roommate to make her living situation financially viable. An older lady with MS (Multiple Sclerosis), who also lived at Gorge at the time, needed similar accommodation. This lady and Michelle were introduced and an agreement was made for them to share the three bedroom unit. One bedroom was for Michelle, one for her roommate, and the third bedroom was for the caregiver.

On September 19, 2002, Dr. D. Clinton-Baker wrote in a Discharge Summary, "The family started work in 2001 and continued into 2002 to find a place for Michelle to live semi-independently. A placement was found and after many months of negotiating and interviewing staff, she was finally discharged from the Gorge Road Hospital on June 3, 2002 to a townhouse on Jolly Place. I will continue from there to look after her."

Moving day for Michelle was very similar to the average person. There was a lot happening. And there were lots and lots of boxes. There was furniture to be placed and the organizing of things into the cabinets. It seemed as if everyone was there to help her: Paul and Cori and Jenn and Tammi and mom and dad. There were also the moving people and hospital staff. It was a joint effort of family and friends. Michelle felt so thankful that she was finally moving into her own place where she could exercise her independence. It was a profound relief to be away from a hospital environment.

Wendy was Michelle's new roommate, a woman in her forties with deteriorating MS. Wendy, with long dark hair, small features, and glasses, had moved into the town house a few weeks prior to Michelle. It was immediately clear to Michelle that this lady was going to be trouble. She was a bit eccentric but, in a meek and timid way, and she was very particular on how things were done. Her expectations of her caregivers were exceedingly high. Wendy used a wheelchair to get around, but was still able to transfer herself from the wheelchair to a chair or toilet. Her oddities would prove to be a challenge for caregivers. They had to deal with her vegetarian lifestyle along with her many food allergies. Wendy's first caregiver, in fact, did not last a week. Family had to take over until another suitable caregiver was found. The problems in this area were often insurmountable.

The situation with Wendy, in Gordon's words: "Wendy was an adult MS patient in the Gorge Hospital with Michelle. About the same time, she needed to get into a better environment and independent living. Those working to make arrangements for Michelle came convinced that the two, Wendy and Michelle, could live together and make a go of it. So, an agreement was reached with Wendy that she would join Michelle in the townhouse and share living and expenses. She would have one bedroom and Michelle another, and then, a bedroom would be available for overnight caregivers. Now, Wendy did not need the level of care Michelle needed, and did not need 24 hour help. She did not need overnight help. So, she hired her own caregiver for the hours she needed and there was no sharing or cooperation between the two with caregiver time. Wendy was quiet, a reclusive person. Costs were hard to determine equitably because Wendy used so little of the townhouse. She stayed mostly within her bedroom. She had some of her furniture, paintings, etc., in the living room. But she was very concerned as to how they got used. Indeed, I remember one time she took some of her things into her room because she feared they would be abused in the open area, living/dining space. She had very particular diets and didn't share at all with Michelle in kitchen supplies; nor preparation of food. So, grocery purchases and things were done completely separately.

"She was disturbed, perturbed and confused when Michelle had dinner parties, or social occasions. She 'hid' in her room and stayed right away so as to not be a part of any such occasions. She usually came out to the common areas of the townhouse, including the kitchen, when Michelle or her caregivers were not there. Quite secretive. It became more problematic as time went on. It left Michelle and the rest of us around Michelle quite uncomfortable. We really couldn't see how it was a very good lifestyle for Wendy. So, in retrospect, it was not a good partnership, facilitated by district staff to enable a solution for both of them, particularly Michelle."

In retrospect, it was a fortunate decision to have separate caregivers, as Wendy "went through" these special helpers rather quickly. It probably didn't help that Wendy was slightly paranoid. Michelle thought the woman was pretty weird when she rearranged the furniture in the living room every time Michelle went away to visit her parents in Kamloops. And Wendy didn't even use the living room. All in all, however, it was a situation that worked. Wendy spent most of her time in her bedroom, only occasionally coming out to use the kitchen or bathroom.

Joan and Gordon advertised in the Victoria Times Colonist newspaper for help for Michelle. They interviewed a woman who seemed to feel she was suitable for handling all of Michelle's needs on a daily basis. She was a small-sized person, however, and soon found the physical demands of lifting and moving Michelle too much for her. Within a week, she quit.

Joan, with the help of Gordon and Sandy, a friend of theirs who was an ex-nurse, took care of Michelle while they continued the search for a new live-in caregiver. Michelle could not ever be left alone without care. When hired help could not be available for one reason or another, "it was a scramble." Joan and Gordon felt bad about imposing on their friend Sandra. Sandra would reluctantly come and fill in, but expressed her feelings that Joan and Gordon were not doing a good enough job of arranging for Michelle's care. It was Sandra's belief that Joan and Gordon should have moved to Victoria to be with their daughter, and not remain in Kamloops. So, when a caregiver let them down, Joan would often have to disrupt her own life and make a "quick trip" from Kamloops to Victoria.

Luckily, they eventually found Robin. Gordon described her as "a most suitable young lady."

Michelle describes the next year as "the closest to a normal life that I've had." Her new townhouse, along with the three bedrooms, had a galley style kitchen that opened out onto a dining room and living room. It had one bathroom that was renovated with a roll-in shower. Michelle had a ceiling lift in her bedroom and later had one installed in the living room so she could be lifted into a regular lounge chair. At this time she was still being fed through a tube.

Michelle and her new caregiver, Robin, "immediately clicked." Robin came from Cumberland, a small community up north in the Cowichan Valley. She had recently finished her certified nurse aid training in Courtney, where she now lived, and was in need of work. On Michelle's 28th birthday, she and her mom and dad drove up to Nanaimo, a half-way point between Victoria and Courtney, to interview Robin over coffee in a restaurant. It was an instant melding of personalities. They called her the next day and offered her the job. According to Gordon, "It was the best thing that happened in terms of caregivers for Michelle. She's (Robin) been such a help to us since, over the years."

Robin began working for Michelle the following week on Father's Day. It was a complicated beginning. Robin's truck had broken down on the Father's Day weekend so, for the first few months, she had to take the bus to work. This involved riding the bus from Courtney to downtown Victoria where she would transfer onto a city bus to take her to Michelle's townhouse. It was a six hour one-way commute. From time to time, Robin would take her 3 children along with her for the scenic bus ride. They would all stay at Michelle's place for the entire week. They had their own bedroom. This would be for four days, as Robin's shift was four days on and 3 days off. And the kids loved it. They were with their mom.

When Robin first worked for Michelle, she was "stunned how much the stroke took from her, how much of her life was gone." Robin thought, "It was very devastating." But Robin was "gung ho and eager" to begin her very first caregiving job. She liked that Michelle was not a "geriatric patient" and that she had all of her cognitive functions. This made Robin's job much easier in that Michelle was totally involved in the process.

After a while, Robin's gruelling commute took its toll on her. She was stressed by being away from her family and how long it was taking her to get home after her weekly shift. When she expressed this to Michelle and her family they came up with a brilliant solution. The Brittons helped Robin lease a new car and offered to make the payments for as long as Robin was working for Michelle. Robin was thrilled. This helped her purchase her very first vehicle. This generous offer by Gordon and Joan also attested to their full awareness of Robin's exceptional qualities. They were very, very pleased with her.

Robin arranged for the children's dad to take care of their three kids, two girls and a boy. She would drive over 200 kilometers, about a 2 hour drive, from Courtney to Victoria, every Monday. She would care for Michelle every day until Thursday, and would return home for the weekend. Joan and Gordon found other caregivers to relieve Robin on the weekends and other special days she wanted to spend with her family. It was an excellent arrangement.

It was initially a bit weird for Robin. She would make up all of her home meals for the week and freeze them. She would then go to work for the four day shift. When she came home, she would do it all over again, make a bunch more meals. The house was a mess, but the kids seemed happy. It would be frustrating for Robin when she would get a call from the kid's dad about a problem. Robin would express, "What? I'm down here. I'm helpless. What can I do? Deal with it." She could sometimes be so exasperated.

It was great that Robin seemed to instinctively know what Michelle liked in regards to her daily care. Michelle liked that her new caregiver was a quick learner. According to Robin, however, it was Michelle who made the entire process easy to learn. "Michelle was good at directing her care." It involved a lot of patience along with a lot of guessing but "it was good because we were so much on the same page." Robin thought that Michelle's use of Morse code was "great." It allowed Michelle to "talk to people." And it was so much faster than the blink board. But even with the time consuming blink board, which was necessary when Michelle was away from her computer, the two young women would work it out. Word for word, blink for blink, Robin would often guess what Michelle was needing, "Do you have the blanket creased under you, or do you have a wedgy", and this would speed up the process. And Michelle didn't mind at all.

Yes, there were times when Michelle "would get defensive" and they would "butt heads once in a while." After all, they spent so much time together. But Robin had the type of personality where she was very patient and would "let things go." She did not take things personally. "It was a pretty intimate time."

The work for Robin wasn't physically hard, but the emotional part could be saddening "because Michelle wasn't getting any better and I didn't know what to expect. I initially had some hope, most definitely. She had some physical improvement in moving her right arm and her leg. Voice, in bed, she would practice more and I was able to understand her better and she would try to say 'dad' and I would encourage her with 'I love you' and try and say my name."

Robin learned quite a bit about Michelle from reading Michelle's diary to her. A lot was explained. Robin felt bad for Michelle: "Her age, how active she was, what she had going on." It was apparent to Robin that Michelle's life had been extremely stressed at the time before her stroke. "I mean, it's no wonder she had a stroke, she was stressed about her weight, getting her coop, her boyfriends, about exercise, just stressed to the max."

Robin sensed that Michelle's emotions had been affected by the stroke. Michelle appeared to have one hundred percent cognition and was totally aware of her condition. There would be outbursts of frustration and despair. Down times would happen more often near the end of Robin's weekly shift as she was preparing to go home. It would be difficult and stressful for Michelle to deal with a new caregiver starting for the week end. Robin "almost gave her an opportunity to do that at least once a week, just have a little bit of a meltdown." Robin would say to her, "It's absolutely devastating the condition you're left in. I don't know how you do it." And then she'd just start bawling her face off.

Some people naturally assumed Robin was Michelle's sister, they appeared so much alike. Robin was a petite blonde with a bubbly, delightful smile. And, similar to Michelle, Robin loved to explore and have fun. They enjoyed baseball games and went to lots of movies. They also took in a few concerts including Blue Rodeo and The Tragically Hip. They loved their many shopping trips where Robin taught Michelle the benefit of thrift store shopping.

Robin assisted Michelle on quite a few trips. She even took Michelle up to Courtney to meet her own family.

One trip Michelle remembered was "great fun." It was to Dome Creek. Robin and Michelle drove in Michelle's van and Michelle's parents followed with their truck and trailer. Paul and Jenn joined them in 100 Mile House. They were all going to celebrate the wedding of a good family friend. The house there was very old, out in the middle of nowhere. There was running water but no electricity, just a generator. Michelle met lots of people and even went on a tractor and wagon ride. She was in her manual wheelchair and could be lifted right into the wagon. One night there was a big reception at the main hall "with lots of dancing and drinking." Paul took Michelle out onto the dance floor. Michelle thought, "I'm in a wheelchair. How on earth can I do that?" But Paul spun her around the floor, teaching her that she *can* do things. Family and friends were very good at showing Michelle to reach beyond her limitations. That night, she danced lots and drank lots. "It's the only hangover I ever got since my stroke."

One aspect of Michelle's care was the handling of the bowels. People pay very little attention to the operation of the bowels, they sit on the toilet, they wipe afterwards. But for Michelle this was something that required more help than merely mother-nature. Robin explained it this way: "Michelle doesn't wear a diaper. You give her a suppository and wait 15 minutes. Sometimes, when it's a shower day, I would put in the suppository, sling her up and put her on her shower chair, she would have her bowel movement, then take her in and have a shower. That's the nicest way to do it. She should get to do that every time. I know she wishes she could shower every day, have a bowel movement every day. We kind of take it for granted, don't we?" When showers weren't readily available, Robin would give Michelle a sponge bath. This was definitely the less preferred method to keeping Michelle clean. And this was how Robin had to care for Michelle when they went on trips like the one to Dome Creek.

Another trip Michelle took with Robin was to visit Cori in Calgary. Cori had settled in Calgary with her partner and his children. According to Michelle, "This was quite a trip." They drove from Kamloops to Calgary in Michelle's van so they could easily get around once there. Robin and Michelle visited the Calgary Zoo, a wonderful place to see all of the animals in fairly natural settings. Michelle, Cori, Robin and Cori's future husband, Chris, all went to a Flames/Canucks hockey game. Michelle, Cori, Robin and Teresa, Michelle's physiotherapist at the Gorge, went to a concert. This was when Michelle met country singer Julian Austin. The weather was nice and they all enjoyed a barbeque outside on Cori's deck. Michelle remembered the only down side of the trip. "The day we left was a horrible snow storm. We slowly made our way through a blizzard to Lake Louise. It eventually cleared up and was even sunny in BC."

Robin would never forget the hockey game. She and Michelle had the bright idea of going outside for a bit of fresh air. It was heavily snowing. But when they tried to re-enter the building, the door was locked. Robin had to push Michelle through a veritable blizzard all the way around to the side of the Saddledome to get in. They thought it was hilarious and laughed all the way. Cori and Chris, however, were not so amused and they complained about the incident. Everyone was amazed when Lanny McDonald sent Michelle a signed Calgary Flames jersey. Robin noted with a smile, "That should be my jersey. I was the one that pushed you."

In August, 2003, Michelle ventured out to witness another wedding. Tammi fixed up her hair and did a beautiful design on her nails. Robin drove her out to Kamloops. The person on this occasion to enter into wedlock was her brother, Paul. It was wonderful for her to see her little brother experience such joy and hope for his future. It was absolutely what she wanted for him. She was so fond of Jenn, his new bride. Yet again, it was a celebration that, for Michelle, included both happiness and sadness. It pained her heart to watch someone else move forward with their life.

It was a marvellous experience for Michelle having Robin take care of her and serve as a fun companion. But all good things, Michelle learned, come to an end. Robin had responsibilities at home. Her partner and the three children needed her. After sharing almost two incredible years with Michelle, Robin had no choice but to resign from her caregiving position.

Chapter 25

Joan and Gordon did not have such tight ambitions for retirement that they felt wrenched out of their future plans in order to take care of Michelle. They were not resentful or upset about that. They simply had a "new regimen" in their lives for the foreseeable future. Some people thought they should have left Kamloops and moved to Victoria to be with Michelle for an indefinite time. Cori strongly felt that way, preferring that her parents be there for Michelle constantly. "However, we had Paul at home, we had a home, and we had a summer home at the Shuswap. And we had a life in Kamloops. Therefore, we did not decide to move, we would commute somewhat. It created some tension for us, because some family and friends thought we would remain in Victoria for an indefinite time."

Michelle found it an unusual experience, being in the position of having to hire and fire caregiving staff. Fortunately for her, most caregivers resigned. But this became a constant challenge for Michelle and her parents. Oftentimes, caregivers simply could not deal with the demanding routine of Michelle's daily care. Some of the caregivers were just not suitable for the job and had to be let go. Others merely did not fit in, due to personality conflicts either with Michelle or her parents.

It was during Michelle's stay in her townhouse that her father pushed for doctors to allow Michelle to eat on her own. She could now swallow small bits of pureed food, enough to ingest a balanced diet. The problem involving medical personnel was the poor results with the barium swallow test. It appeared to the doctors that Michelle could not swallow properly and was in jeopardy of choking. It remained hospital policy that Michelle be tube fed. However, according to Michelle, the tests were not accurate. During the test she would get nervous, thereby not able to relax enough for proper swallowing. After all, how many people experience difficulty swallowing while nervously sitting in the dentist chair? There were a couple of other things that interfered with Michelle's swallowing during the test. She was sitting up straighter than usual during the test, and she was also given smaller bites than she normally dealt with.

It was clear to Gordon that his daughter could do quite well eating on her own. The one thing that Michelle did not lose from her stroke was her sense of taste. This meant she could enjoy one of the most pleasant sensations in life, the sweetness of ice cream, a perfectly seasoned mushed up hamburger, a thickened, ice cold beer. It was a battle for Gordon with the medical system to allow this simple pleasure for Michelle. After time, however, he convinced doctors to give the "okay" to mouth feeding. A household blender became a very useful kitchen appliance in Michelle's home. It was another step in the direction of Michelle's having as normal a life as possible.

• • •

David Edwards was Michelle's next caregiver. He had been employed at the Gorge Road hospital when Michelle first met him. So, it was nice that she already knew him. His looks had changed since she had seen him at Gorge. At that time his hair was dark and thinning. Now it was shaved right off. He was quite good looking, with the most beautiful long eyelashes. She liked Dave. He was a divorced guy with a couple of kids he had at home on the weekends. He lived close by to Michelle's place, so he would sometimes have her over for dinner and a movie on his big screen TV.

Dave liked to take Michelle outdoors. He was tall and thin, but very strong and easily handled Michelle in her manual wheelchair. Victoria offers a good variety of wilderness trails and bicycle paths. One especially fun excursion was up to Sooke Pot Holes. Dave pushed Michelle in her wheelchair up a gravel road, and then pushed the chair over the mossy ground through the trees to what looked like an old train stop. Then they went through the trees again to a half built wooden lodge. Apparently the building was meant to be a resort, but the owner ran out of funding, so there it stood, unfinished. Michelle absolutely loved the adventure of being within nature. She had missed it so much. "It was beautiful."

The adventurous side of Dave's life appealed to Michelle. They would go to the outdoor adventure store where Michelle took a keen interest in the various items displayed for outdoor living. She was with Dave when he purchased a river kayak. Dave and his girlfriend, Cathy, went kayaking and camping together. For Michelle, watching the relationship between Dave and Cathy develop over the years was hard. Michelle knew "that will probably never be me."

It was very good for Michelle to have Dave in her life. He was strong enough to lift her and place her in her chair in the living room. It was close to normal, sitting in a chair other than a wheelchair. All of the outdoor hikes on bumpy paths seemed to be strengthening her neck muscles, and this allowed her to sit up on her own for longer periods of time.

Once again, however, Michelle had to endure another change in her life. Dave suddenly resigned.

Michelle's next caregiver was Rob. He had begun as Michelle's weekend caregiver and was willing to become full time. Michelle considered herself lucky because Rob was a personal trainer. With Rob's help, Michelle lost a bit of weight and grew stronger. The two of them did something almost every day. One time they went to the beach at Sooke. There was a huge dead tree trunk lying on its side on the beach. The roots of the tree were exposed and were quite high. Rob hung Michelle's lift motor on these roots and was able to lift Michelle out of her chair and onto the beach. Michelle lay on the sand and smelled the salt air, "and the fresh sea air was great."

Another time Rob and Michelle went camping at Windermere Lake where Cori and her family had a summer trailer. Michelle liked that Rob was big and strong and could handle looking after her in a tent using a floor lift. She had her commode and shower chair with her. This was a combination chair that usually stayed in Michelle's bathroom. It had a mesh back and a black seat that was like a toilet seat, only softer. When it was discovered that the showers there were inaccessible, Michelle was wheeled into the lake for bathing, even though body-washing and hair washing was really not allowed.

Michelle recalls, "Rob was really a great person to know. He really believed in tough love. He often left me to struggle to do something myself which might seem mean but really gave me a sense of accomplishment." Michelle also noted about Rob, "I remember going for a walk on Dallas road and stopping to do some leg lifts. It was great motivation to have some eye candy. He wasn't big on clothes so it was often shorts and T-shirt and sometimes in nice weather just shorts."

Michelle very much enjoyed talking health with Rob. They had discussions about diets and exercise and metabolism. All through Michelle's life she had been concerned with health and weight, so her and Rob had quite compatible beliefs. It wasn't always perfect. Michelle had her stubborn ways and Rob had a bit of a temper. This made them "butt heads" from time to time.

Rob had no qualms over taking Michelle out in public. He once took her to a strip bar to watch a football game. It wasn't the first time Michelle had experienced this type of bar, and she felt quite normal being there. Michelle felt Rob was a benefit to her "overall wellness." She was very happy with her weight loss and became more mobile, gained more confidence and "grew that thick skin again."

• • •

Cori and Michelle decided they should travel to Mexico. Cori booked a one week Air Transat holiday in the month of November to Puerto Vallarta. Rob and Richard, a weekend caregiver, went along to help Michelle. They were joined by Cori and her boyfriend, Chris. They all met in Vancouver for their flight. It was Michelle's first trip since her stroke and she was very excited. She loved airports and planes. She was in her manual chair and was rolled up to the plane door. Rob and Richard lifted her into the airplane seat. Michelle had her computer with her for communication, but "Rob could read me well and I didn't need it."

Upon arriving at the airport in Mexico, Michelle was strapped into a narrow airplane chair and two Mexican men from the airline carried her down to the tarmac and into her wheelchair. It was a pretty unnerving time for Michelle. She had severe vertigo which could be terrifying, so she just stared at the sky, praying for the ground to soon be under her. Part of the holiday plan was for Michelle to have a wheelchair accessible van. Unfortunately they were provided with just a regular van with no access for a wheelchair at all. Michelle had to be lifted by her two male caregivers and placed onto the bench seat of the van. She had to lie down all the way to the hotel, so she saw nothing of the drive through the streets of Mexico.

The group of them stayed in an all-inclusive resort in Nuevo Vallarta, just outside of Puerto Vallarta. In the bathroom was a bathtub, not the roll-in shower they had been promised. The floor was terracotta tile with a drain. This was where some creativity was involved when it came time for Michelle to shower. Using a standard manual hotel wheelchair, she was placed beside the toilet, resting her head on the back wall. The first time they tried this, they flooded the room. Michelle thought it was hilarious. Rob tracked down housekeeping and was provided with a large squeegee to clean up.

When they went down to the beach the guys lifted Michelle into a lounge chair. It was such a great time for Michelle, taking in the warm weather, admiring the glistening ocean, and, her favourite pastime, people watching.

The guys worked very hard for Michelle. Whenever they went anywhere they had to lift her wherever the wheelchair would not go; down to the beach, up staircases, and over questionable terrain. One day they did manage to get a wheelchair van and drove into Puerto Vallarta. They walked downtown to an outdoor mall and market. Michelle noticed black and orange flags everywhere. At this market was a rickety swinging bridge they all had to traverse. Michelle was intimidated by the wooden planks that were missing some boards in several places. The market was stretched out along the bank of a river. It met up with a boardwalk way above them that ran all along the beach. Rather than walking back the same way they came, Rob and Richard decided to carry Michelle in her wheelchair up a very, very long flight of cement stairs. It was a lot of exercise for the guys. For Michelle, it was an exercise in trust.

The restaurant at the resort set aside a special table for Michelle. Each day the guys would take turns pureeing her food in her little blender right there at the table and spoon feeding her. Each evening they all went out to the main patio to meet the other resort guests and take in the nightly entertainment.

Michelle's most memorable part of her vacation in Mexico was swimming with the dolphins. Her entourage travelled in the same wheelchair van to an animal compound where there was a large building with a souvenir shop and a set up for bookings for the dolphin encounter. Michelle sat outside under an umbrella at a round table while Cori handled the paperwork. When this was done, they headed down a cement road to a general meeting area. Here among about thirty other people, they were introduced to a gorgeous parrot. From there they all went down to a nicely finished wooden shed that had televisions and open windows. They viewed a short program about dolphins, then peeled off their clothes down to their bathing suits and donned blue life jackets.

Michelle had been wearing a sarong across her lap and legs that was easy to pull off. In a way she was lucky. Because of her disability, she had a separate pool and her very own dolphin. Rob and Richard lifted Michelle from her chair, sat her on the edge of the pool, and gently eased her into the water. Michelle was "in awe of this intelligent, cute bottle nose dolphin." Michelle's left side was mostly paralyzed and, somehow, this dolphin could sense this. The dolphin delicately pushed at Michelle's left side, helping her to move. It was an amazing experience that Michelle would never forget.

On the flight back home, Michelle and one of her caregivers were bumped up to first class, which was a nice bonus. Michelle had taken a shower after her swim with the dolphin, but her body still had a definite fishy smell. Getting back to her daily routine was "such a let-down." When she took her next shower, there was a hint of the dolphin odour. It was a nice reminder of a very special moment.

Rob was with Michelle for quite a long time, about 14 months. Michelle considered him her favourite caregiver. In the fall of the year Rob resigned after taking on a job at a hospital north of Victoria in Nanaimo. On occasion, he would come back to take care of Michelle, filling in for a couple of days when her other caregivers needed some time off. In the future, no one would ever quite compare to Rob.

Joe, her next caregiver, was a fellow who was experiencing problems with his weight and was actually working with Rob on a training program. He lived in Nanaimo, but didn't mind the drive to Victoria to take care of Michelle. During Joe's eight month employment with Michelle, he lost a lot of weight, a testament to Rob's good training. Michelle liked Joe, but she very much missed Rob.

When Joe left, Michelle's next caregiver was Jen. She had a cute little baby that she brought to work with her. The baby was so good. Michelle was happy when watching a baby. She wanted to hold it, snuggle into the baby's soft skin. She wanted to play with the tiny feet while changing a diaper. She craved to tickle the baby's belly and make it burst into happy little giggles. But instead, she could only watch.

Chapter 26

It was time for Michelle to move on. Finding reliable caregivers in Victoria was becoming very difficult, and besides, Michelle was in need of a change. She had never been one to grow roots in any one place. One of the main reasons Michelle decided to move off the island was her fear of the entire island sinking into the ocean from a major earthquake. Actually, this was not altogether an unreasonable thought. Vancouver Island is located on the "ring of fire," the well-known circular zone where most of the earth's seismic activity has occurred throughout the history of the world. And Michelle had experienced one of these quakes while lying in bed one morning at the Gorge Road facility. The earthquake shook everything for quite a few seconds. Michelle recalled how helpless she had felt at the time.

There were a few other reasons Michelle chose to make a change in her life. Yes, staffing difficulties was a huge consideration. Michelle, not unlike a business, had to deal with all sorts of employees. There was the variety of odd personalities, the assortment of caregiver's family problems, the constant actions of irresponsibility and, occasionally, problems with substance abuse. However, Michelle's need to be closer to her parents on the mainland was her main priority. Even though she had a strong desire for independence, the close proximity of her family would definitely be a comfort. And she did realise they were the only ones she could fully trust.

There was one other aspect to Michelle's relocation quest. Rob, her most favorite former caregiver, had parents who lived in Kelowna, a city situated in the Okanagan Valley. If Michelle were to live in this area, there would be a good chance she could see him more often. This was very important to her.

So, this is where Michelle moved, to the interior of British Columbia, specifically the stunningly beautiful Okanagan Valley. The Okanagan is well known for its tourism. Okanagan Lake is the main attraction for visitors from all provinces of Canada along with lots of tourists from the United States wanting to experience the vast beauty of the lake and the area's wonderful warm summer temperatures. And the lake is definitely vast. It is large and deep. It spans and area of 135 kilometers in length and 4 to 5 kilometers in width. It has a surface area of 351 square kilometers. Its maximum depth reaches down 232 meters. Okanagan Lake is home to several species of fish including rainbow trout and kokanee salmon and, of course, the legendary but elusive lake creature, Ogopogo.

Kelowna is the largest city in the Okanagan Valley, situated on the narrowest part of Okanagan Lake. The city has grown to a population of 115,000. It is easy to travel to Kelowna. It is 400 kilometers from Vancouver, 600 kilometers from Calgary and a mere 150 kilometers from the US border. Positioned in a valley between low mountains, Kelowna has some of the warmest temperatures in the country, averaging 80 degrees Fahrenheit, or 27 degrees Celsius in July and August, perfect for enjoying local parks and beaches. And, for Michelle, it was favorable that Kelowna was a mere two hour drive to her parent's home in Kamloops, just close enough, but not too close.

In downtown Kelowna, located near the corner of Ethel Street and Guishichan Road, is a healthcare facility by the name of Cottonwoods. It is described as a residential care home that provides residential care and specialized geriatric services. In Joan's view this was not the proper place for Michelle. Residents there were mostly elderly people who were experiencing various health problems that were leading them towards the end of life. Because of the change in location for Michelle, from Vancouver Island to the Interior of BC, she lost her funding for independent living and had no choice but to move into Cottonwoods "temporarily" until a more suitable residence could be found. She would live there for "five long months."

To Michelle, Cottonwoods was an "old facility in Kelowna with mainly old residents." And for a person who so much hated hospitals, this place was "too damn close."

In Michelle's semi-private room her roommate was a "crotchety old lady that kept us entertained." Sometimes Cori would come for a visit and bring her cute little dog. Well, the old miserable woman absolutely hated dogs, so staff would attempt to distract her from seeing Michelle's four legged visitor. Sometimes they would hastily shuffle the old lady right out of the room. Michelle didn't really know what was wrong with her old roommate and, frankly, didn't care. Maybe the woman was in her eighties, although Michelle figured the woman's gruff demeanour most likely made her seem older than she actually appeared. It was guessed that the aging woman suffered from dementia, but Michelle didn't think she was all that bad and "was still walking."

Even though Michelle hated Cottonwoods, hated being in an environment of the sick and dying, she did have some very good experiences there. She met all sorts of wonderful people: doctors, physiotherapists, caregivers, social workers, support people, occupational therapists, and volunteers. Michelle had met some "really great people since my stroke that I never would have met otherwise." They all did their best for her. She would be put through a general range of motion regimen in bed twice a week. And she had regular physiotherapy in the Kelowna hospital rehab centre. The Cottonwoods facility bus would transport Michelle to the hospital where she would receive her therapy and HandyDART would drive her back to Cottonwoods. Her physiotherapy at the hospital involved standing her upright and putting her through exercises of turning her head and lifting her arms. She was also fitted with new foot splints to keep her tendons from shrinking.

One person Michelle met while staying at Cottonwoods was Arlene Pilgrim. Arlene worked for the BC Paraplegic Association. The objective of the BCPA was to provide support in all aspects for people with spinal cord injuries. That would include everything from health to transportation, accommodation, sexuality and employment. Initially the focus of the association was on new injuries, but Arlene found herself working with all people with spinal cord injuries, both new and old.

Arlene was contacted by Michelle's BCPA consultant in Victoria who told Arlene that Michelle had just moved to the Kelowna area. The Victoria consultant explained a little bit about Michelle, how she had suffered a stroke and was quadriplegic and had lost her speech. Consultants with BCPA were trained to engage with spinal cord injury clients, even if they did not ask for help. It was the purpose of BCPA to make sure clients knew consultants were available if needed. So Arlene went to visit Michelle in Cottonwoods.

It was a professional requirement for BCPA consultants *not* to express sympathy for their clients. They were strictly there to help. Arlene did find herself curious about the details of Michelle's stroke. Arlene found it odd that such a young person with no pre-existing conditions and no indication of health problems had experienced a stroke. She was surprised that there was no high blood pressure and no record of strokes in the family history. It just happened. Arlene could not ignore the fact that Michelle had just gotten started with her working career after graduation.

One of the main things Arlene wanted to do for Michelle was "to get her out of Cottonwoods." The frustrating part for Arlene was that Michelle was "in the Interior Health system" and there were procedures to follow. Arlene could see that Cottonwoods was not the most favourable environment for a young person. The patients were mostly seniors. Alzheimer's was a prevalent condition there. The rooms were very sterile and "hospital-like." Arlene had to leave the problem of relocating Michelle to be handled by Michelle's nurse case manager and her social worker.

Arlene did try to do some research in finding Michelle a better computer because hers was very slow. She contacted everybody she could think of in Vancouver to see if there was anything faster. She saw in some research that there was a computer that was operated through head movements. But everything Arlene found that could be an exciting improvement for Michelle required a certain degree of eye and head movement. None of the new gadgets would work for Michelle.

There was definitely some success when Arlene searched for someone to drive Michelle's van and take her out places. Arlene contacted Kelowna Community Resources, along with some senior's places. That's when she found Les. He also had a disability, cerebral palsy, but he was quite mobile and could handle most physical tasks. Actually, it was Les who initially approached Arlene, looking for some volunteer work to do. Arlene suggested he drive for Michelle and he took on the responsibility of getting her out and about. Arlene thought "he was really good with her."

Arlene did her best to help Michelle get in touch with various organizations that helped her regain a certain level of outdoor activity. The organization, People in Motion, introduced Michelle to Powder Hounds, a skiing group up in Big White Mountain Resort. Powder Hounds offered unique skiing and recreation opportunities for physically and sensory challenged individuals. Michelle, using a neck brace from the hospital, finally renewed her love of skiing. It was "really nerve-wracking" the first time. Michelle's vertigo was still causing her an extreme fear of heights. Going up in a ski chairlift was daunting. Her dad and the ski instructor sat on each side of her, protecting her from visualising how high they were. She did just fine. They placed her in a special skiing sled and scooted her down the hill. She would partake in this activity every winter from then on.

A bonus from Michelle's renewed outdoor adventures was the strengthening of her neck muscles. It came to the point where she needed only a soft collar for skiing and no collar at all for hiking. Through her new connections, Michelle discovered the CRIS (Community Recreation Integration Society) recreation group. She could go hiking using a special chair called a Trail Rider, which was something like a canvas wheelbarrow with one wheel. All she needed was someone who could drive her van and, of course, push her along in her Trail Rider.

This was when Michelle came to depend on the generosity of volunteers. It was a good thing that she met Les. Michelle liked him. "Les was a really good guy. Good sense of humour." He was often available to take her hiking or to do other things, such as grocery shopping or banking. There was one time he had to take her to emergency when her Gtube (for feeding) fell out. Even though he had cerebral palsy, she could see he was high functioning. He could talk and was able to drive. "He just walked a bit funny, with a knock-kneed limp." It was nice that their hiking took Michelle into areas she would otherwise not have the chance to experience. She loved the sweet earthy smell of the woods where she could "reach out and grab tall grass." There was a bit of a downside, however. Even though Les was very helpful and considerate and had that great sense of humour, he was overly protective of Michelle and tended to "treat me like I didn't know better." This, as with anyone who did not respect Michelle's intelligence and independence, sometimes annoyed her.

The operation of getting Michelle into the van and properly securing her chair could be an intimidating process for some. There were a few people who, although qualified to take care of Michelle, just could not deal with the complications of operating the van and its many gadgets. Michelle's vehicle, the Dodge Grand Caravan, was equipped with a folding metal ramp at the side door. It was not a power ramp. When the door was opened, the ramp was manually lowered down, first one section, then the other. Michelle's wheelchair just barely fit on the ramp and had to be carefully guided on or off the vehicle. Once Michelle and her chair were inside the van, she had to be steered to the front passenger side where the seat had been removed leaving a generous space for the wheelchair. Michelle could help in the process by using the wheelchair power to roll the chair up completely to the front. There were tie down straps in the front of the chair along with some rather frustrating attachments that slid into some slots in behind on the floor. If a person was not used to the contraptions, it could definitely be a mechanically demanding procedure.

For those who were able to manage the physical and technical aspects of taking Michelle out, there was unfortunately the fear of dealing with her precarious health condition. Michelle was dependent on someone to make sure she was comfortable in her chair, that a cloth was placed between her head and the headrest, that her arm was properly positioned on the armrest, that her hand could reach her devices for operating the wheelchair, that her computer was placed in front of her on top of the support tray. For Michelle's family, who were accustomed to all of this, it was nothing more than a daily task, but for those who were new to the world of a quadriplegic, the intricacies of handling Michelle were unnerving.

Consequently, it was nearly impossible to find a person who was willing and able to take Michelle out to do the simplest things, such as going for a stroll in the park, shopping at the mall, or going to a movie. Not only did Michelle have to find someone who met all the criteria in handling her, but also a person who could spare the time from their own personal life. It was not easy.

One very nice person Michelle met through the BCPA was Jo, the executive director of Lifestyles Equity. Jo took interest in

Michelle's desperate desire to move into a more homelike environment. This company had a few homes that housed the disabled, providing staff and a van. Michelle and Jo became friends.

One of their first outings was to a presentation of a UBCO nursing class. Michelle laughed when Jo first tried to feed her. Jo was feeding Michelle thickened red wine and was doing just fine in Michelle's opinion. But poor Jo, like all new people with Michelle, was tentatively gentle. Michelle "told her not to be so ginger." Michelle thought it was funny.

Jo did lots of things with Michelle. She invited Michelle and Cori over for dinner a couple of times. Jo lived with a wheelchair bound roommate, so her place was wheelchair accessible. One dinner was a fancy potluck dinner party where two people were in charge of the main course along with the appropriate wine. Michelle loved it. It seemed so…normal.

Jo and Michelle would also go out to a movie once in a while, and even to a pub. Jo tried to help Michelle arrange Michelle's birthday party at a pub called YukYuks. It was a shame that nobody showed up. It seemed that Michelle had not yet developed close and reliable friends in Kelowna. But Jo and Michelle still enjoyed the party along with the chocolate cheesecake Jo brought from Tim Horton's. That evening, it was a weird and entertaining experience for Michelle and Jo to sneak back into Cottonwoods after nine. Everybody was already in bed. "It was like a ghost town."

Finally, after enduring month after month at Cottonwoods, Michelle's "team" found for her a much better place to live, Mountainview Village. Once again, Michelle was on the move.

• • •

Arlene Pilgrim had tried her very best in finding ways to improve Michelle's daily living. It was mainly Arlene's tireless efforts that kept Michelle in touch with organizations such as CRIS, an offshoot of People in Motion. The main drawback for Michelle to take part in different activities was her dependency on volunteers. And a huge problem was funding the costs for someone to drive her places. Arlene "turned every stone" trying to find some money for Michelle, "but there was nothing."

Arlene was surprised by Michelle's ability to cope with her disability. It was obvious to Arlene that Michelle was "very frustrated." What really impressed Arlene was Michelle's ability to maintain a good sense of humor. Arlene remembered a time when she attended an information session with Michelle put on by staff of GF Strong. At the meeting there was a beautiful buffet lunch. Arlene was impressed that it was so well organized. The food smelled and tasted wonderful. But Arlene felt sorry for Michelle. There was poor Michelle, stuck eating this pureed "goop." And she was being fed by Arlene, and Arlene at best was incompetent. Similar to others who have tried to take care of Michelle, Arlene was terribly afraid she would choke her.

The one thing Arlene says about having a spinal cord injury is, "If you get hurt, get hurt on the job, or in a car accident." That way, in Arlene's opinion, at least a person would have proper funding through the government or from a financial settlement to carry on a better life. People like Michelle "don't have that."

Chapter 27

Mountainview Village was an assisted living building with one section for younger people. Each person had their own suite. Michelle was fortunate to have her own bedroom, bathroom, kitchen and living room. It made her so happy to first see the suite. She even planned a small party, even though she had not been in Kelowna for long and didn't know too many people. She invited some folks from Cottonwoods and they sat around the living room talking, eating, and drinking. Michelle ate spinach dip and hummus. Whoever happened to be sitting beside her would assist in the feeding. She also took part in some drinking, rum and fruit juice, or red wine. For the most part, Michelle's involvement with her friends would consist of her listening and enjoying the good conversation. Sometimes, someone would sit right beside her and engage her in a private talk. I was very refreshing for Michelle to once again take part in a normal friendship gathering. The quality of her life had improved so much.

This was one of the things that Arlene first noticed about Michelle. When Arlene visited Michelle in her suite, all the leftovers of the prior night's party were there, scattered dishes and liquor bottles. Arlene thought it was quite funny. Here was this young woman with extreme disabilities carrying on with life in a pretty normal fashion. Arlene was definitely impressed.

Living at Mountainview gave Michelle an enormous boost in her self-esteem. She had very much regained her independence. She was able to email doctors and friends. She made contacts with all sorts of people. She ventured out more often on the HandyDART. And she also had a driver for her van, so there were so many more opportunities for her to go out and explore life. And she didn't stop at just the one dinner party. She had her own personal space where visitors could come and see her without feeling like they were in a hospital. It was so much better.

Michelle had returned to an environment where she was receiving a lot more help with keeping her in good physical condition. In regards to better physiotherapy, Michelle recalls, "Sabine was my physiotherapist in Kelowna. She had an English accent and was very helpful. It was in the rehab unit at Kelowna General Hospital. From Cottonwoods I took the Cottonwood bus and at Mountainview village I took the HandyDART there and back. I spent some time lying or sitting on the plinth. Sabine had an assistant, Jon, who mainly did my physio on a tilt table. Once I was upright (on the table) we did arm and head exercises. I really felt this was helping. I could lift my right hand and shake Jon's hand."

Michelle explains some of her therapy. "While I still had physio I had another round of serial casting. It was a tough stretch but I wanted to do it. Eight weeks of hell. I drank lots. Heather, Heather and Shannon were from the community. Heather was the boss of Heather and Shannon. Twice a week I had about forty five minutes a session of range of motion, stretching exercise. Heather started and then had to take maternity leave so Shannon took over. After about a year at Mountainview I lost any real physio. I had new foot splints and the ROM stretching. Now I have lost a lot of flexibility and dorsiflexion."

Terje, the pastor at Mountainview, was able to drive Michelle's van. Terje, Michelle, Derek, and another resident would all visit different parks around the city where they would have a picnic. Or, sometimes they would just go for a drive.

Jo was the one who would help Michelle out with her dinner parties. Sometimes Jo would cook, and sometimes Michelle would make her famous chilli, with some of Jo's help, of course. There was always wine and good conversation. Derek, a resident and Michelle's friend, was a humanist and didn't believe in God. Terje, on the other hand, was very strong in his religious faith. Even though they respected each other's beliefs, they couldn't help, in Michelle's words, "getting to it" from time to time. This was very entertaining for Michelle.

When Michelle had been in Mountainview for about a year, Cori got married. The wedding took place at Windermere Lake, near Calgary, where Cori and Chris had a summer trailer in Shadybrook Park. Michelle, along with her parents and Jo, drove Michelle's van out to the lake and stayed at a bed-n-breakfast. Paul and Jen, with their new 3 month old baby girl, went out separately, and stayed at a nearby motel. Everybody gathered at Cori's trailer for a barbeque dinner. Michelle always thought it was a weird family dynamic when they all got together. Cori would give most of her attention to Michelle while their mom and Paul seemed to disappear somewhere. Most eyes, of course, were on the baby. Michelle thought it was good for her to see people in a regular environment, and it was also good for people to see her in a normal situation.

The wedding was a simple outdoor ceremony. They were lucky with the weather, the rain holding off for a while. Pictures were taken before everybody moved inside the community hall. The reception was typical, an entertaining slide show, lots of drinking and dancing. Since her stroke, weddings became one of Michelle's least favourite things. It was a time when she would "have to watch a normal couple very much in love looking forward to a life together and probably with kids." It was a cruel reminder to Michelle that she would most likely never have this experience in her life. She was happy for Cori, yet once again, could not resist feeling sad for herself.

Michelle did make another attempt at dancing in her wheelchair. And she discovered she could actually meet guys at a dance, even though they only gave her a few crumbs of awkward attention after they were very drunk.

• • •

After the wedding, Michelle and her parents went back to Kelowna where they spent some time visiting. About a week later, they all drove out to Vancouver to catch a cruise ship to Alaska. Michelle was so excited. They were all prepared with her shower chair and a portable lift. Michelle's former caregiver, Robin, would join them on the cruise. She met them in a large white warehouse building where they registered for the cruise. They were ushered upstairs through an area resembling an airport terminal. This is where they went through a customs check. Paul and Cori and their families were already boarded, however, a computer problem caused Michelle and the others a bit of a wait. During this time, Michelle got caught up with Robin, who she hadn't seen in years.

Finally they were led through some doors to a switch back ramp up to the ship. Once on board, Michelle was amazed. She thought it was very classy. It had large paisley carpet, two theatres, a casino, a spa, an indoor pool, and some outside hot tubs. A suite was set up for Michelle's disability, and she and Robin shared the room. It had two twin beds, a love seat, closets, and a roll in shower to accommodate Michelle in her wheelchair.

Breakfast and lunch were served in a large buffet cafeteria. Staff on the ship blended any food Michelle wanted. They were very helpful. Dinners were more formal. They dressed up in skirts or suits before going to the dining room. A three course meal was served with liquor, wine and coffee. All of Michelle's food was nicely pureed. Cori and Robin took turns feeding Michelle.

Each night, right after dinner, they would head into the theatre to enjoy a different show. Robin and Michelle ventured into the casino one time and were thrilled; they won ten dollars. Then they ventured up to the nightclub. Once in a while they could feel the choppy sea. There was a scary incident one evening with the swaying boat. Robin and Michelle were going back to their room after some time at the casino. Robin had not been drinking alcohol; however, it certainly appeared that way. The two women were making their way down the hallway, Michelle going all over the place in her chair, with Robin staggering right behind her. Once in the room, Robin hoisted Michelle up in her sling, getting ready to place her into bed. Suddenly the portable lift swayed sideways and Michelle was helplessly swinging in the middle of the air. Robin quickly steadied the pole, and nicely saved Michelle from a hard landing on the floor.

Their first stop on the cruise was Sitka. The ship anchored in the bay and people were taken to shore on small boats. Michelle was unable to go because of her wheelchair. She didn't mind not going into Sitka. She knew there would always been certain things she could not do. She was content to remain on the ship and go to a movie with her mom and dad, *Happy Feet*. Then they explored the ship and took in the sights of the Alaskan landscape. Michelle noticed that, even though it was August, the air was quite cold.

Michelle was happy for Cori's stepchildren. They had lots of freedom on the ship. They could go off on their own, using walky-talkies to keep in touch with their parents. There was so much for them to do, including a pitch-n-putt and a rock climbing wall.

At Skagway the whole family took a train ride up the valley. One of the cars of the train had a lift for wheelchairs, so luckily Michelle was able to go along. It was a great trip; the train ambled up the side of a mountain that framed the valley. It was a beautiful, sunny day that showed off the river and gorgeous wildflowers growing everywhere. They went past waterfalls, old bridges and old unused tracks. It was so wonderful that, of all the things Michelle had lost in her life, she had not lost her ability to explore the world.

And sometimes having a disability had its advantages. The captain was fascinated with Michelle and her use of Morse code on her computer. He invited her up to the bridge to watch the glacier 'calving.' It was quite the experience, with the thunderous noise of the ice breaking off and plunging into the water. And Michelle was very impressed with the bridge where the blue carpet and blue wood walls made it "very regal and official looking."

One thing, in Juno, was "really neat." The bus was equipped with a metal box compartment sized to fit a wheelchair. The wheelchair was driven into the box and then the box was lifted by hydraulics until the wheelchair was at the same level as the other passengers. Michelle was impressed by this new technology. When they arrived in town, they spent most of the day shopping. Michelle's impression of Juno was, "It is quite a tourist Mecca."

She quite enjoyed her time on the ship. The main lounge was located in the ship's centre. Michelle thought it was a great meeting place. There was a bar and a dance floor. Michelle and her party often had drinks there. To look upwards was magical, especially at night. It was all lit up. All of the balconies on all of the floors looked down upon this lounge.

It was a wonderful trip. It was so nice for Michelle to have every moment of her day filled with excitement and joy. But, like every dreamlike vacation, this too would come to an end. She headed back to Kelowna, back to reality. It was a shock for Michelle to "adjust from one caregiver close by to easily and quickly help to waiting for a care aid to even answer the call bell." But after a day she settled into her routine and "it's like you never left."

• • •

Robin had joined Michelle many times, as a caregiver, on vacations. They had travelled to Calgary for the Stampede and a hockey game, to Dome Creek for a wedding, to Vegas for shows and gambling. And Robin even helped out Michelle in Vancouver when she had a few weeks treatment in a hyperbaric chamber. But of all the travelling situations they had experienced together, Robin thought the cruise was the very best.

Chapter 28

It was simply not in Michelle's nature to stay any one place for very long. She spent almost two and a half years at Mountainview, but became generally unhappy with the place. For the most part, in truth, her spirit became restless. In Michelle's view, "nothing felt like home."

She thought it might be better for her to live in Vernon where her brother, Paul, and his family had settled down and bought a home. Both Paul and his wife, Jenn, had begun their teaching careers. Their little girl, Emery, brought much joy to Michelle; however, it was not easy for Paul and his family to travel to Kelowna that often. It was important to Michelle to be close to family. In Vernon she would even be a bit nearer to her parents, reducing the drive to Kamloops by 30 minutes.

She began searching for a new place to live in Vernon. It was her plan to apply for CSIL funding in that city. The rule was that a person actually had to be living in the city where they applied for this financial assistance, so Michelle had very little choice but to seek out a complex care facility in Vernon. This would be a major step down for her in regards to her independence.

Michelle made a few trips to Vernon to check out a couple of facilities. One was Heron Grove; another Creekside Landing. Her final choice would be Creekside Landing. It was a brand new building and had no waiting list.

Everything happened surprisingly quickly. When managers of Mountainview discovered Michelle was looking to move to Vernon, she was placed on a list that gave her thirty days to move out of Mountinview. Michelle says, "Little did I know that things were going on behind the scenes."

Michelle wasn't sure who, or what organization, was involved with pushing her so quickly out of her Kelowna residence. She was certain that "They heard I wanted to leave and took the opportunity to get rid of me. Apparently I was too much work for assisted living and I gave them an easy way out."

Before she knew it she was living in Creekside Landing. Even though it was a state of the art facility and very nicely designed, it was still basically a complex care facility that did not at all give the impression that people living there had one bit of independence. Michelle had one room with a bathroom. That was it. She did not like it. She lost the freedom of having her own large space. She lost her privacy. In the last four years she had gone from living in a townhouse, to an assisted living suite, to one room. She was very bitter.

On her first day in Creekside Michelle met Mary, an older lady who instructed in arts and crafts. Mary was instrumental in helping Michelle learn to paint with limited control of her arm and hand. A sling was devised to support Michelle's very weak right arm. With this help, Michelle could hold onto a paintbrush. Mary would move her arm to specified areas of the canvas, and Michelle would paint small landscapes.

Mary "innocently" printed some of Michelle's paintings onto blank cards, and a small business began. Michelle hired a friend to help her set up a website for her where she started selling prints, cards, and calendars.

Now that she was at Creekside Michelle had to satisfy herself with the simpler things in life. Her room had a south facing window that nicely displayed the main entrance and circular driveway of the complex. Michelle loved to watch staff leave from the main kitchen door that was only about ten feet away from her window.

She would sit in her usual spot between her bed and the bathroom and watch people come and go, observing life beyond the confines of her small room. Depending on the type of day she was having, this pastime of hers could bring forth feelings of happiness and contentment or sadness and regret.

But Michelle's life still included her greatest love, travelling. After a few months at Creekside she and Cori and some other ladies all went to Las Vegas. It was a girls' trip. It was a fun group including Michelle's mom and a family friend around her mom's age, along with Robin and her own mom.

Michelle still loved flying. Getting her aboard the airplane was a bit of a chore. She and her caregiver were allowed to board first, going through the process of dismantling her tray from her wheelchair and removing the computer. Michelle was then lifted from her chair and placed into a narrow airplane chair that could be wheeled down the aisle. The chair did not fit very far into economy class so Michelle had to sit in the first row. It was at this time that Michelle realized she must "really watch my weight."

The first thing Michelle noticed about Vegas was "it's so warm." Another thing she noticed that really impressed her was how wheelchair assessable the city was, even offering a wheelchair taxi to the hotel. MGM was fantastic, with a bellman at the covered front entrance, "like in the movies." Once inside they were immediately struck by the din of clanging slot machines. Michelle immediately noticed the giant screen behind the front desk advertising the different things to do in Las Vegas.

She and Cori shared an upgraded suite. It was "amazing." The main living area contained a chair, table, phone, lamp and sofa with a coffee table situated in front of a large TV. On the other side of the sofa was a large dining room table that really came in handy. A door led from there into a large bedroom with a chair, another TV, and a nice king size bed. From this room another door led into a large, long bathroom that stretched the full length of the suite. At the end was a very convenient roll-in shower.

Michelle described Las Vegas this way, "I love this city."

Robin was Michelle's caregiver during this trip, but she only dealt with Michelle in the morning and at bedtime. The rest of the time Michelle was with Cori. The sisters visited an outlet mall and the Paris Hotel. They spent some relaxing time at one of the five pools in the MGM Grand Hotel.

A highlight of the trip was the show Thunder from Downunder: male strippers. Michelle thought it was a real classy strip show, although she admitted to not having seen too many of these types of shows to allow for much comparison. After the show they did the typical tourist thing, having pictures taken with the "guys" and purchasing some souvenirs

The next day they packed up and flew home.

Michelle was suddenly thrust back into her daily life. She had difficulty describing what it was like there at Creekside, the atmosphere that surrounded her. It wasn't all entirely bad. A wing of the home was set aside for youth, that being residents under 60 years of age. Initially there were only four of these young people. They were taken out to movies on occasion and were escorted on shopping trips. They were involved in a special supper club and did this once a month.

Michelle did her painting once a week. Thankfully, she would have visitors once in a while. And her friends and family would come as often as they could and take her out, oftentimes for an entire weekend. To Michelle these times were like breaking out of prison.

But for the most part Michelle's days were, to put it bluntly, boring. She described them as, "Get up, email, TV, lunch, email, TV, dinner, email, TV, bed."

Over the months she did her best to improve the quality of her life. After about a year of waiting for some kind of action on

getting into a more suitable place to live she sent letters to various government organizations in an attempt to acquire assistance.
This is her letter:
To Whom it may Concern:

My name is Michelle Britton and I'm looking to change my current living arrangements. Currently I am 35 years old and have a commerce degree from the University of Victoria. I was born in Kamloops and lived in Victoria when I had a spontaneous arterial dissection which caused a stroke.

I suffered a stroke 10 years ago while living in Victoria. I was just finishing a business degree from UVIC when I suffered a brain stem stroke after a terrible 5-day migraine. I spent about 6 months in acute care at Victoria General Hospital before moving to extended care in the Gorge Road Hospital in Victoria. I was now quadriplegic and couldn't speak.

While at the Gorge Road Hospital, I went to GF Strong in Vancouver for 7 weeks to learn Morse code in order to communicate via computer and voice box, and to get accustomed to a power chair. I was in the Gorge Hospital about 2 years and another lady and I moved into an accessible townhouse with SCIL funding. I was able to have 24 hour care. This really was a wonderful arrangement. However, after over four years it became very difficult to find reliable care staff. With my primary proponents (my parents) living in Kamloops, I decided that it was time to move to the interior of BC.

After five ugly months at Cottonwoods Hospital in Kelowna, I moved into an assisted living suite in a "young people's" wing at Mountainview Village. That always made me laugh because at 32 years old, I was the youngest resident; all others were over 40 years of age. My intention was to stay in Kelowna while I explored CSIL options in Vernon, where my brother and his family live. That didn't happen and I was put on the Access list, having no choice but to move to Creekside Landing in Vernon. That was over a year ago and I am still in Creekside Landing.

I would like to live independently and not feel like I am being tucked away in a Seniors Residence to dwindle away the rest of my life. I understand the baby boom population is growing and there is a definite need for more facilities; however, what about group homes for young disabled people? Why aren't there more group homes? There have been many group home closures and others my age have been forced to live in a Seniors Residence as well. In the last two years, I have lost the privilege to physiotherapy and since living at Creekside, I worry about my health physically, mentally and emotionally.

Since moving to Creekside Landing over a year ago, I really have lost a lot, both physically and mentally. I lost physiotherapy while I was still in Kelowna and now I only get the "range of motion" exercises. I am losing flexibility and dexterity, both of which I need to carry on sitting in my power wheelchair all day keeping my own head up and to be able to use my right arm and hand properly in order to operate my computer (imperative for my communication to others). I used to go to the symphony, theater, or even a pub or two in order to maintain a "normal" young person's life. Here, at Creekside Landing, I am unable to do any of that as the night staff cannot put me to bed any later than ten pm (there is no staff on after ten o'clock who are qualified to do so). In fact, I don't get out much at all anymore.

The rules here are developed for the older citizens and persons with dementia living here, not younger residents such as myself and a couple of others. We are just supposed to follow the rules; there are no legitimate discussions with us to find out how we feel about our living arrangements. I grew up as a strong able-bodied person and now that I am physically unable to do things for myself, it seems I am given rules that limit me even more. No one should live like this, without some hope for a somewhat "normal" life, feeling useful and respected by others around them.

I know the Interior Health Authority is different from the Capital Health Regional District. I just don't understand why it is so different or why it has to be different. Does each region have different resources? And if so, why? I really think there needs to be a closer look at where the resources are coming from and where they are being dispersed. I would like to know why I was able to have all I needed to live in my own home with 24 hour care in Victoria, but I am unable (so I have been told) to have that same arrangement here in Vernon (especially when Vernon is the city where my family lives, not Victoria).

I realize that you may be quite busy these days, but would there be a chance to meet with you in person? You would understand how unfair my situation seems, to meet me in person, as I am a vibrant, young, charismatic individual who has so much to offer my community. If given a chance and given hope of an independent life while being useful to others, you will see just how much good will come of this meeting. I really wish to create a movement for all those young persons in Vernon and the Interior who are in the same predicament as me. There is so much I have to offer!

Thank you so much for your time and consideration. I hope to hear from you as soon as you have a moment. The best way to get a hold of me is by email at:

Sincerely,

Michelle Britton

c/o Creekside Landing, Vernon, BC

• • •

One letter from the Social Planning Council seemed encouraging. It reads as follows:

Hi Michelle,

Thank you for your email and being willing to share your story with us – it sounds like quite the journey for you and your family. I admire your determination and perseverance. ..

I've done some research to see what housing is available to a younger person with a disability. Unfortunately, it seems this is definitely a gap in our community and that the only assisted living available to younger people is through the network of senior's complexes. There used to be a society called the North Okanagan Handicapped Association that provided assisted living that was not just senior focused but they have since closed their doors and sold their two group homes. The Vernon Native housing Association does manage units that are wheelchair assessable and designed for people with disabilities, but they do not provided any supports.

The Mayor, Ms. Baumbrough, and I are a part of the City's Affordable Housing Committee and will bring up this issue at the next meeting. I know this won't help your immediate situation but it will ensure that this gap is addressed in future planning. In the meantime, I'm wondering if you know about a society called Independent Living Vernon (previously known as the Vernon Disability Resource Centre). They're a great resource for getting connected in the community and also have programs for assisting with employment, volunteer opportunities and resources for starting small businesses. There number is…and website:….. The Vernon Native Housing Society contact number is….

I wish that I could provide more immediate help Michelle but I really do appreciate that you contacted us. Your story has definitely made an impact and I will be advocating for addressing this gap at future planning meetings for housing.

Sincerely,

Annette Sharkey

• • •

Other agencies sent very brief, non-committal letters to Michelle. One of these letters reads partially as follows:

I have done some research regarding your housing situation and unfortunately your situation falls under Provincial jurisdiction. I note you have sent this e-mail to your MLA as well so I will leave this matter in Mr. Foster's hands.

Yet another letter says, in part:

My name is Kristen Keill. I am the Office Assistant at Mr. Eric Fosters MLA Office. He asked that I look into your concerns regarding your living arrangements.

Upon my contact with Kari Hedstrom at Interior Health she has informed that she has been involved with yourself and family in regards to this matter. She would like to continue dealing with this issue directly and has requested that you contact her. Kari is the Patient Care Quality Officer for the North Okanagan. She has been very helpful in the past so I advise that you continue to stay in contact with her.

I will be closing this file on my end but if you require anything further or are not satisfied with the outcome, please contact me. Thank you for taking the time to write.

It is curious how most agencies that sent a reply to Michelle thanked her for taking the time to write to them, as if she was living a busy, full life and managed to squeeze in a bit of time out of her hectic schedule to write them. It seemed such an obvious contradiction to her complaint.

• • •

During Michelle's stay at Creekside she ventured out to Coquitlam, part of greater Vancouver, for hyperbaric therapy. Cori helped Michelle with the organisation, hiring a caregiver, and arranging the actual therapy. The idea of HBOT is to increase oxygen to the brain to help stimulate and regenerate cells. It was very expensive therapy. Michelle was fortunate in that several people, including family and friends, donated to her cause.

Robin would be her caregiver during this month long experience, so that made Michelle comfortable. She really enjoyed spending time with Robin. Michelle thought this adventure was "truly weird." It was "right up there" with some of the crazy things she had done in her life. And Michelle very much believed in this alternative therapy. To her it was better than taking a bunch of pills.

The therapy involved transferring Michelle onto a wooden spine board and sliding her into a capsule onto a vinyl bed pad with cotton sheets. She was sat upright and pivoted on her "butt" until her right shoulder was on the softer surface and Robin would lay her down and adjust her to a comfortable position. After a ten minute wait for the chamber to pressurize, Michelle would remain inside the chamber for one hour breathing 100 percent oxygen. For this hour she would "think and think and think."

There were 40 of these sessions altogether. Michelle would think, "Is it going to be worth it?" She was bored and tired. After one week of treatments she hadn't really noticed any change in how she felt physically. She was sleeping better, unsure if this was due to the treatments or because she was just tired. Her parents were flying to Venice that day. Michelle wished it was her going there. She wanted to see Venice. She wanted to see everything.

After three weeks Michelle still felt no change. She really wondered why she was doing it. Then she began laser treatment, which was part of the program she paid for. Michelle was amazed at how the body reacted to the laser. The neurons in her body almost immediately responded, making it easy for her to lift her right arm. The left side of her face was tingling, as well as her left arm. She was amazed how the laser could trigger tingling in both her face and her arm at the same. She was very happy with the results.

One of the best parts of the entire experience of her HBOT was meeting a new friend. Gary was having therapy for a rare brain disorder called "executive disease" that was attacking and shrinking his brain. It was fortunate for Michelle that Gary also lived in Vernon. Gary, a medium sized fellow with strawberry blonde hair, had been a successful man, owner of a larger auto dealership in the city of Vernon. He even had his own place in Hawaii. But his condition had deteriorated to the point where he had to sell his business and retire.

After they both returned to Vernon upon completion of their therapy, Gary visited Michelle about once a week. This was a wonderful new addition to her life. Since his oxygen therapy, he seemed to have no change to his brain. And this was a good thing. He had seen many doctors and there were various theories and diagnosis', the latest being Lyme disease.

Gary figured out how to email Michelle from his cell phone and proceeded to email her every day. He vacationed in Hawaii for several months through the winter, but when he returned in the spring, he visited Michelle almost every day. Gary got himself a Bouvier puppy and named her Kona. But this was no ordinary dog. Kona was trained to be a service dog and would be there to help Gary if he had a seizure.

What Michelle liked about Gary was his charm and good sense of humor. He was the latest of the many wonderful people she had met over the years.

• • •

For most people, moving from one home to another, although often stressful and challenging, is a relatively simple task. Sell the house. Give notice to the landlord. Send out change of address notices. Pack up, and move. The entire process normally involves no more than a few months.

With Michelle, this same goal would prove to be a major test to her patience. She tried everything she was capable of doing. Most times for her it was like hitting a brick wall. There was just so little in the "system" for her. Programs and funds were drying up all over the province. But Michelle pressed on. Overall, her plan took four years.

• • •

Presently, Michelle is once again in her own place, living independently. To her credit, she single-handedly sought out financial resources that would support her daily needs for independent living. She hired a realtor, researched the real estate market, and, with assistance from her brother, Paul, went out and looked at various places until she found just the right one. Cori was the one who purchased the townhouse and Michelle pays her monthly rent. It is a perfect situation.

Daily care still presents a bit of a problem. Michelle is only allotted funds to pay for nine hours of care per day. She is still working on acquiring more. Michelle's safety is a considerable worry for her family. However, she has a bell set up that will dial a couple of people who can assist her in case of emergency. During the daytime, should Michelle need help, she is able to contact friends and family via email or texting. Cori has accepted Michelle's need for independence and has told her sister she will absolutely not carry any guilt if something should happen to her. Both sisters are content.

Michelle's living space is a two bedroom ground level bungalow apartment in a very attractive complex. There has been an automatic door-opening system installed above her front door so she can, with the push of a button, open it for visitors. There is a very nice modern kitchen with light oak cabinets and stainless steel appliances. The main living area has lovely dark laminate flooring, which could easily fool the eye into believing it is expensive solid hardwood. There is a large window in the room that displays the front patio and a pleasing distant mountain view.

Along one side of the main room is a full sized couch with a lovely set of ceiling to floor wave design mirrors on each end of the coral coloured wall. Right opposite is a nice new while wall unit where Michelle has stored trinkets, photos, books and an assortment of videos and CDs. There is also a brand new flat screen television. Both the wall unit and TV were gifts from Michelle's new friend, Gary.

Michelle's bedroom is nicely set up with her special bed and the appropriate lift equipment attached to the ceiling to assist caregivers in getting her in an out of bed. There are also two bathrooms in her condo, one a smaller bathroom for her guests. The larger bathroom has been renovated to Michelle's needs. The floor leading to the shower has been gently sloped upwards to allow for her wheelchair to roll right in. It is perfectly designed. Now Michelle can have a shower whenever she chooses, as long as there is someone there to assist her. The second bedroom has not yet been painted, but will be set up as an art studio, so Michelle has a place to pursue her artwork.

It is a wonderful, comfortable place. The walls are Michelle's colours. The air inside is as fresh as the outdoors. Michelle's determined adventurous personality is understood when one sees the tiny gecko ornament displayed on a shelf, the picture of her swimming and laughing with the dolphins, the collection of photos from travels all over the world.

But most of all Michelle's condo simply looks like an average regular place, for an above average and above regular person.

Michelle is home.

Chapter 29

Everyone has a different perspective when it comes to thoughts of Michelle's incredibly rare circumstances. Each of Michelle's family and friends has expressed personal views that were thoughtful, emotional, and often surprising.

Sandy Fulton, the first social worker to deal with Michelle in the ICU and Neuro sections of Victoria General Hospital, remembers when she helped Michelle with acquiring her Broda chair. "It was a beautiful purple chair, you know, all fluorescent, like a car with a beautiful paint job. It was pretty high tech. It would help her do a lot of different things that our chairs couldn't. It was a very good chair."

Sandy was impressed by the family. "That they were always realistic that things may not get much better than they were at that time. But that was okay with them. Being realistic, they maintained hope for a future. They always thought that Michelle would make some gains, not 'way out there' but some gains." And Sandy was so happy that Michelle had made quite a life for herself. "She's going skiing and she's going hiking and doing all this stuff that's fantastic. And she's making connections in the community as well. She's building her network, which is really important."

Sandy, like most people, went into deep thought when considering how she herself would have dealt with such a severe disability. "Oh Lord. Well, my kids already know and so does my husband that if certain issues come up...That's when you get into a really tricky question. If there is no hope for recovery what the heck does that mean. Meaningful for Michelle and her family may be different that it is for me and my family. If you can have a quality of life, then I think, okay. If you are going to be in a vegetative state, which Michelle isn't, but there was a fear that she would be, if you're going to be in a vegetative state, then is that what you would want for yourself? Probably not. I was in a family conference once and the physician said to this family, 'if your person can no longer choose what they want to eat, what they want to wear, who they want to be with, where they want to be, do you think that they would want to survive?' And I put that into my own practice because quality of life is so important. Michelle has a quality of life from what you've told me."

Adele Schroeder, Michelle's childhood friend, looked at Michelle's situation, not from the perspective of her profession as a medical doctor, but as a young woman who valued the quality of her life.

"I would like to believe that all things happen for a reason; that God has a master plan for each of us, which, though it may not be what we desire, has some greater purpose. I say I would *like* to believe that because it would make things so much easier. Most of the time when I think about what Michelle has gone through since her stroke, the path her life has been forced to take, the future that isn't what it should be, I am just angry and sad. Even after all these years I can't understand how her life is supposed to be like this. I don't know how she has such strength and courage to face each day and to face it with the same smile I remember from growing up. I don't think I have ever told Michelle any of this. How do you tell your childhood friend that you don't think you'd have the strength or will to go on as she has? My visits with Michelle are usually for an hour or so once per year at Christmas when she is in town visiting her parents. Conversation is awkward as the slow, monotonous computer interpreter speaks for Michelle. Sometimes I find I end up having a conversation 'around' Michelle rather than 'with' her.

Her sister or parents provide answers and anecdotes on her behalf. It makes things easier at the time, but afterwards I always feel a bit guilty. Guilty what I struggle to have a regular two-way conversation; that I never made the short drive from my home in Kamloops to hers in Vernon for a visit; that I have a husband, children and career; that I can walk, talk, sing and dance. Yet I have never once heard Michelle express self-pity or anger towards her situation. Through all the frustration with the logistical side of her journey: the fight for more physiotherapy, for better communication devices, for assisted living that meets her needs as a young person, she has never given up or given in but has persevered with courage. I admire her so much.

Michelle still has the same genuine smile and every time I hear her laugh her physical inabilities disappear and I am reminded that the real Michelle is unchanged. And I am blessed to call her my friend."

Jason Clappison, the young Australian fellow who spent time with Michelle on her travels, has his own unique perspective on Michelle's complicated life. His own path in life was very successful. He acquired his Engineering Degree and, after a brief stint in the Army Reserves, joined the Electrical Design Engineering Group at GM. He takes great pride in being one of the two engineers that designed the "fuel sender system for the home grown Holden Commodore auto. He moved on to the mining industry where he currently works as a Project Engineer.

About Michelle, Jason says, "Independence was one of Michelle's stronger attributes although she was never overly forceful. She had ideas and things she wanted to do and see but if she couldn't do it today, she'd do it the next. She was very considerate. I do think about Michelle quite often and she's never too far from my thoughts….I think her turn of events are tragically unfair. I wish science had developed to such a stage as to be able to give her life back, even if just a little to begin with. I know the technology will be there some day, and just like Michelle, I want it here now."

Arlene Pilgrim, who helped Michelle through BCPA, the British Columbia Paraplegic Association, has possibly seen too many people with disabilities fall through the cracks. Her view is, "I would not want to live like that. She (Michelle) had everything to live for, her age, her education. One thing about Michelle, she did a lot of living before the stroke, so it's a good thing. I would wish I had money to have all the supports."

Paul Britton, Michelle's brother and most nearby relative, is very supportive of his sister. It is obvious that he loves her dearly. He reflects on past and present events: "There was a sense of resignation, but the progress from a vegetative-like coma to her ability to recognize and acknowledge you was a relief and any twinkle of her eye or smile she could muster was worth its weight in gold. I loved trying to make her laugh when I visited her. I remember being so proud of my sister when she went across the stage in a wheelchair to received her Business degree that she had completed just prior to her stroke."

Paul comments about coping with Michelle's ordeal: "There is no formula or manual to deal with this type of grief and it took me a long time to sort out my emotions around this. There was a weird mix of guilt, sadness, depression, and thankfulness that each took its turn driving the bus. I think that it wasn't until my daughter, Emery, came on the scene that I really gained clarity on those emotions and was finally able to end the grieving process. The bottom line is that my big sister is still with us and I need to treat her like my big sister. I don't do her any service by feeling guilty, pity of sad about her lot in life and I give her more service by treating her like my big sister, my friend and auntie to my 2 kids. I owe Shell her self-respect and her independence in any way that she can (sometime I probably push her a little hard in the independence area but it's what I would want for someone to do for me). I won't let her give up on her fight…And it's important to recognize that it is her fight and I can't own or wear that. Having 2 children of my own has also given a new level of compassion for what my parents experienced. The thought of that happening to my kids is enough to make a man crumble and beg for mercy or sell his soul in exchange. I hope that I'd have half the strength my parents did in dealing with the crisis at hand."

Robin Campbell, Michelle's caregiver in Victoria, has known Michelle for many years and keeps in close contact with her. They are close friends. Robin is very outspoken about the needs of a person like Michelle. "I loved working with just one person. I don't call it spoiling, but I could take very good care. Going from what she had in Victoria to what she was getting in Vernon; so much time is spent alone and I think, ugh."

Robin speaks about Michelle's time in her townhouse in Victoria and Michelle's parents: "I love them. They felt terrible that they couldn't be there but they also had their own lives, right. They felt bad and if they were absolutely needed to be there they would be there. It might take a little longer; one of the caregivers would have to stay a little longer in order for them to get there. The time when I was with Michelle there were actually not times when we couldn't deal with it ourselves. They weren't required to be there for any emergencies. Michelle had some pretty unreliable…caregivers."

Robin offers an opinion on Creekside Landing, the Vernon care home Michelle wound up living in for four years. "I think it's sad. I mean, yes, she says that the caregivers she has are good and they do what they can. I'm sure it's just like one of the manors we have here (Coquitlam). Absolutely amazing, just top of the line, but the care just isn't there. At least where she is now there are some younger. There's quite a bit of drama she's expressed. I just find it sad. Why is the opportunity not there to live within assisted living, do what she had on the island? Why can't she do that in the interior? I wanted her to move here. I kind of justified it because the airport was here and she could just fly to Kelowna. The valley, as far as accessibility goes, stinks."

When asked how she herself would deal with having such a severe disability, Robin says, "Not very well. I'd want to do what Beanie (a man with paraplegia) did and numb myself so I didn't have to feel the…I think it would be a different story if I didn't have children. I'd probably not want to live anymore. But having kids that would probably give me some…I'm hoping that's what Michelle's friends and family help her with.

Kristy Gregson, another of Michelle's childhood friends, has stayed in contact with Michelle over the years. Kristy remembers: "For several months, while she (Michelle) lived there (Victoria), I visited Michelle in the Victoria General hospital. She learned to use the alphabet board (I am not sure of the proper name of it) to communicate. So, one blink was 'yes' and two blinks was 'no'. That was exhausting for Michelle, however, it was her way of communicating and by having some say it was her way of having some control in her life. Michelle was mentally all there, but locked in. I felt so bad for her every time I went to visit. Also, I missed her voice and her laugh and had hoped for years that it would return. I continued to visit Michelle during her time in Victoria. She was later moved to the Gorge Road Hospital where she lived for a few years before moving into subsidized housing and having caregivers look after her. I still did my best to visit Michelle in person, but also stay in touch with her through email. As the years passed, I found it more difficult to visit consistently…got married…teaching full time…(and family problems)…I felt really bad and guilty that I couldn't get over to see Michelle regularly like I had before, but she understood that life got busy. Although I knew that Michelle was very frustrated with her situation, she was very understanding and was just happy to see me when I got over to see her…Michelle was a bridesmaid in my wedding in 2001. Michelle looked radiant and she had a lot of fun that day, as did we."

Kristy reflects on Michelle's life: "I feel very sad for the way Michelle is living her life…not able to walk, communicate, work, or lead a normal life, etc…like she so very much deserves. I find that Michelle is much more structured and serious than she was prior to her stroke. This makes sense in that she doesn't want to lose control of her life and wants to have a say in her life. Her computer is a vital tool for her to communicate with people. I feel Michelle has some very strong inner strength that has been getting her through the years. She was always a believer that 'things happen for a reason'. Her artwork is also something Michelle enjoys doing. I am so grateful that Michelle has a supportive family who spends time with her, assists her with decisions, etc…Michelle is a dear friend to me. If I had one wish, it would be to hear her voice and contagious laugh again."

• • •

Tammi Henderson turned out to be one of the most loyal and consistently helpful of Michelle's friends, especially in the days, weeks and months of Michelle's stay in Victoria General. Tammi reflects on the first thoughts she had about Michelle's future. "I honestly didn't think she would not walk again. And I didn't think she would never talk again. That's been the hardest thing for me. You know, you want her to be her again. But, you know what? She still is her, just a different Michelle."

Tammi gained a new perspective about disabled persons. "Well, her and I joke around a lot when we go shopping and people just walk right in front of her and I think, you know what, 10 points for every person you peg because this is just ridiculous. So that is just kind of an ongoing joke for us, like, every time we go out. And I admit that I was one of those people when I was growing up, and of course you look and go, woo, what happened to that person, I mean, I don't even know how to respond to it."

When Tammi remembered the time she spent in the hospital with Michelle, Tammi was emotional. "I didn't worry about her dying. She's just one of those types of people that has a very strong personality and, there were times when she and I would be talking and she would break down and just say I can't do this anymore, so I just kind of talked her down and said, 'You know what, you're doing amazing so far. I know that it's not your life that you had before but we can do so much more with you now.'…No, it's good to talk about it. It's not an unhappy cry."

Tammi talked about her ideas about Michelle's possible recovery. "I didn't know because, like I said, we didn't get any answers until probably a couple of weeks, it felt that long to me anyway, until they actually found out it was a stroke she had, and what type of stroke it actually was. And only five people have been noted to have this so, I'm, well, leave it up to you to do that, you know. She says, I know. Like, I love her to death, I do, but, and the thing with me is, like, every time this stuff happened I would get a phone call and Tammi would come and talk to her she's not having a good day and I was just one of those people that would just go up there and make her laugh, having problems at the hospital, and it was just non-stop. I didn't know what to expect and, you know, when you started hearing voices, sounds coming out of her throat, like, go, do it, and then it didn't happen, but with her whole left side not working, I thought, okay, well there's therapy, we can just work on it. I actually helped, I was with some of the physiotherapists watching them do stuff with her but I didn't know when it would happen.

I was an optimist. I wanted to see her walk again. I think her parents hadn't been around her for a period of time, I don't think they knew who Michelle was, because even Cori and I think along the same lines of who Michelle was, or is, and her parents didn't. And it's just because she was kind of the black sheep of the family and we all knew that and everybody still knows that. She led her own life and she did her own thing and that's just who she was."

When considering if she now thinks Michelle will ever get better, Tammi says, "No. I know she'll never walk, I mean, she had to tell me. One part that is really hard for me is that I moved away from her, I moved to Jasper for six months and I didn't want to move but it was just a job…but the week that I moved was the first week that they got her to stand, and I missed it. That was very, very hard for me. Her muscles and her hips and her upper body wouldn't support her to stand so they didn't know what else to do. And because it affected her left side so much, like her legs work and that's what shocked me the most, both her legs are fine, just her left arm, it's basically asleep for the rest of her life. It's basically, her arm is sleeping; it will sleep for the rest of its life."

It was difficult for Tammi to come to terms with Michelle's inability to walk. "Well, it's just been recent for me. I still kind of felt that there is still something that they could do as long as they found some person to do physio on her or somebody that would take the time. That's been an ongoing problem. I even said to her, I might as well just go to school, be your caregiver for the rest of your life because this is ridiculous, and then I said to her I don't want to give you a bubble bath because I'm your best friend and we just don't do that. But that's just the way our relationship works, if I could be there to do stuff with her and know that I would be fine with paying my bills and doing that sort of stuff and she wouldn't have to look for somebody else, I would do that, but then it would get to a point, okay, what's more important to me, me looking after her or my friendship with her, and my friendship with her is more important than losing that because something would happen between us."

It was Michelle who finally convinced Tammi that walking again was probably not going to happen. Tammi says, "I think the biggest thing for me was when she told me; that's heart wrenching because I want to see you walk again. She just kind of came to terms, like, you know what, I'm never going to walk again, and I know in her eyes, and I know in her mind, and as much as she thinks that I don't, I do know her, she probably didn't want to hear that ever in her life because of who she is."

Tammi does not think of herself as someone special. "I think because Michelle and I had such a close relationship, we were really good friends, because something like this happened, never want to say sorry, I don't want to be friends with you because you're different. She's not different. She might be in a wheelchair. She still has an amazing personality. She has a great sense of humour. She's Michelle, it's just you have to deal with her differently now. And not in a bad way, it's just making yourself trained to be something different, and it's a learning thing for me and that's what I thrive on is learning new things and I still love her, she's my best friend…I don't care that she can't talk and I don't care that she can't walk. She's still a person that I can talk to and she can talk back to me. She's 100 percent all there. She even remembers everybody's birthdays. She knows when she did this. She remembers phone numbers still from people that I don't even remember from when we lived in Banff. She's 100 percent there and that's the thing that probably shocks me the most is that her mind is 100 there and her body is so affected."

Some people say they would rather be dead than live like Michelle. Tammi thinks, "I would never say that I would want to be dead, but you know I always think to myself that Michelle is probably one of my heroes. I don't know how she deals with the stuff she deals with. I think I would probably have given up quite a while ago. Like I said, I would never want to die. I would want to live and live my life the way she's been doing it. Absolutely. Travel. Do as much as you can. Figure out how to make yourself get to the point where you want to be. She travels more than I travel and I try to travel but... But, you know what? I think she's done amazing."

Tammi comments on Michelle having to live in an institutionalized environment. "She's a nomad. And that's just who she is.

That's her personality. She was a traveler. She wanted to do everything. I think the house she had in Victoria was ideal for her cause it was her own place, then she moved to Kelowna and got put into this home. And the whole thing with her is that, she likes to have a shower, have a bath. It hurts me that she had to go through that, all the time, and I know that she's been accustomed to it and she's over it, but at the same time, I don't think she really is, but she shouldn't have to live in environments like that. She's still young. She's not an old person."

Finally, Tammi says, "I think she's going to accomplish everything she wants to accomplish in this life."

• • •

Jo, Michelle's friend whom she met through the Lifestyle Equity Society in Kelowna, has some very interesting thoughts about Michelle, her condition, and the way society handles her. "When I met her (Michelle) in Cottonwoods we clicked right away because I knew she knew. I could see people around her being condescending and she and I right away got that immediately…and we'd laugh… and the people would come in and talk in a high voice to her and we'd look at each other…you know people were yelling and it's like, she's in a wheelchair, she's not deaf. She was really tongue and cheek about it."

Jo had a good feeling about Mountainview. "Then she moved into Mountainview which was a wonderful place. She had her own apartment. She had some good friends there. The only down side was…they didn't provide for going out into the community. It would be nice. I would go over there and cook dinner and bring wine and I'd just thicken the wine and spoon feed her wine and I'd drink wine."

Jo describes Lifestyle Equity Society. "We served people. The movement was always about community. Not group homes. Group homes are stigmatized. I used to say to staff, 'Do you want to live here?' If the answer is 'no,' then…we better pull up our socks. "

"Generally," Jo continues, "I would go over and I would bring the food and cook and we'd have dinner. Sometimes we'd have dinner parties with Terje the pastor, Derek a guy who lived there, and Michelle and I. We did this maybe three times and we would have so much fun, drinking and eating. Michelle does fabulous, but it's because the three of us would just get carried away. She's taking it all in. Once you know Michelle well, she really understands humour. She's sarcastic. You can't really see the brain injury."

Jo speaks about extended care. "There are some nice people in extended care facilities but it is a system, for starters, where funding is an issue so there is not enough staff to do the work. From my perspective, I don't believe anybody, I don't care how old you are, should ever have to live in a place like that because my belief is that if you can breathe, you are entitled to a quality of life. It's congregate care. It's stinky. And there's people dying all over the place because it's full of old people and no young person should ever live there. I think it's a system. People in there are very much institutionalized, like the staff, like they don't have the vision. It's about dollars. It all comes down to dollars. It's a more cost effective way to serve people…it's dismal."

Jo has an enlightening way of looking at how people with disabilities should be able to live within society. "Mountainview is assisted living, there's a variety of people there. All kinds of people. And they all have some kind of health issues or something that they need support. It was a really good place. I'm not into anything with conjugate care. It's like ghettoizing. You have all of these people with some type of disability, all living together; it's a very segregated environment. It really is. I have judgements about any building that's full of disabilities. Some of the stuff that Community Living has done is they'll take an apartment building and they'll have five people with disabilities living in units throughout the apartment so that each person is seen as their own person and so they get to know their neighbours around their unit. If 10 percent of the populations have disabilities, then an apartment building should have 10 percent of people with disabilities. Not 100 percent. Because that becomes a segregated environment. Mountainview was fabulous, striking a balance. Although everyone has some type of need, the units allow for individuality. It is a great compromise. I didn't get that sense of the nursing home."

Jo speaks sadly, yet hopefully about Michelle's life. "Michelle blows my mind. I think she's amazing. Her tenacity…and she never gives up. I feel bad that I'm not a bigger part of her life. The loneliness is probably really tough for her and having people around her who really get her. I think that's probably one of the biggest frustrations. Her family's dead on. They're amazing. They're completely respectful and they treat her just like another member of the family…and so did her friends."

Jo wonders how she herself would deal with such a severe disability, saying, "You know it's funny because I've asked myself, would I be able to deal with it like Michelle has dealt with it. And I think the fact that I'm a mother and grandmother…but I think those are the things that give me a reason to want to be alive. We in society put so much value on stuff. It's about mobility and what you do and how much money you make. It makes us a valuable person but, when we truly examine the things that are important to us, it's friends, it's relationships. It's sitting and being with people. Those are the things that bring us happiness and joy. In knowing that, I would like to believe that I would start to really look for those moments rather than giving up because I can't walk anymore. A human *being*, rather than a human *doing*.

• • •

Scott Guthrie, the man Michelle may have one day married, remembers how he felt when he first heard of Michelle's long term diagnosis. "I can remember her dad explaining to me what had happened, the Spontaneous Arterial Dissection. I remember talking about the symptoms she had in the days and weeks prior to the incident. 'Incident:' that is what her mom and dad tagged it. It was now known as *the incident.* I do not remember where or when it was that I learned of her fate and what her life was to be like when she woke."

Scott's love for Michelle was reflected in his thoughts when he learned Michelle may never walk or talk again. "I have to get back to Victoria and be with her. I need to help her through this. I need to move back and be a part of her life and offer myself to her."

For quite some time, Scott needed to be with Michelle. "For the first couple of years after her incident I was trying to find a way back to BC to live. I had applied for a compassionate transfer with the military to move back but was denied because we were not married. I tried an occupational transfer to another occupation but that did not work. All I wanted to do was return to BC and be with her. Despite my efforts it did not come to pass. Then, over time, I began to move on and live again, dating and going out with other women. At which time I met my (present) wife."

If Scott had married Michelle before she had her stroke, his life would have gone in a totally different direction. "Am I happy we are not married because of her disability? Not at all. I think I would have adapted and we could have shared a great life together. It would have been extremely difficult but love conquers all and we would have been just fine. However, life turned things in a different direction and I am happy that I have the family I have now. Had I married Michelle my life would have been very different and I can't imagine my life being different than it is now."

One last thing Scott mentions is a testament to his love for Michelle. "I actually have a picture on my desk from that trip. Nothing more than a picture out the side of the aircraft looking out over the clouds. It is quite beautiful and a nice reminder of the time I spent together with Michelle."

It is imperative for a father to provide for and protect his children. For Gordon Britton, his need to give Michelle a good life is evident:

"For me, it's meant much regret. Regret for Michelle's changed life. Not for myself. What life would she have had if not for this medical intervention? For me, there's been a tension throughout the years between abandoning our independent life for Michelle's needs; or maintaining much of our intended retirement.

"At the outset, some, Cori included, believed we weren't involved enough. We should have 'mothballed' our life in Kamloops and have been constantly with Michelle in Victoria. We weren't confronted directly with this view, but sensed it in little comments made by those around us, including some friends. And, yes, there are those we know who did give up their independent lives for the care of a loved one. We argued (mostly with ourselves) that we could not just suddenly give up our home, relationships of 30 years, our son Paul's needs (he was still in Kamloops). However, the examples of others who DID just that were out there. Anyway, we made the decision to try to do both; give Michelle support and maintain the thread of our lives.

"Then, there is the question, why did this happen to a bright, beautiful, 24 year old? There were those who suggested it had a purpose. It would challenge her to respond to life differently; be inspired to deal with her disability and be an inspiration to others! Nonsense, not sensible. No, no spiritual, pre-ordained reason for her medical incident. Just plain accident: a weakness in the artery in the brain. No rhyme or reason for me!

"People have frailties and ailments but then look at Michelle and how she's coping and feel their problems are diminished by comparison.

"So, there is always regret that Michelle could not have a regular, full life."

Joan's thoughts were a bit different that her husband's. "As a parent, we always want the best of lives for our children. With Michelle's incident happening just before her 25th birthday and starting her career with her Bachelor of Commerce Degree in Tourism, it was devastating to all our family and friends. Our family and extended family rallied around and brought us all closer together. There was a lot of stress from the event put on the family as we travelled our own journey with our relationships with Michelle. Dad and I trying to remain strong to support Michelle, Cori and Paul. Michelle was and is a very strong person and gave us lots of encouragement. As a mother, I wasn't angry at the event but at times despair would set in, and grief. Grief especially at her cousins' weddings soon after as I realized Michelle would not have one herself but she just enjoyed the moment for those getting married. She's been bridesmaid and is going to be maid of honour for a very dear friend in the fall.

"Michelle has given many folks encouragement through her life and they see their lives could be worse off. I know Michelle gets frustrated with people who are not willing to help themselves to a better life and that gives us comfort in that she is being positive herself. She has developed many friendships with her cheerful attitude and self.

"Michelle is a determined woman. She is looking forward to living independently with care help. Her family is very important to her, especially her younger niece and nephew who love her. We try to give her pleasures in life, for example, trips to Calgary, Alaska (cruise), Mexico, Las Vergas. She comes to Kamloops at least once a month, or Shuswap Lake a couple of times a month in the summer. We find love and happiness is especially important in life as one never knows what is going to be dealt us in the future."

Cori's views on Michelle's life are thought provoking and inspirational. She comments on how she felt about Michelle's misfortune: "I have very little anger about her tragedy. I feel frustrated at things like the Ministry of Health or bureaucratic hoops to jump through to get some basic things for my sister to try to give her an independent life because she is young and vibrant and shouldn't be in a senior's residence. I get frustrated at people who don't take her emails seriously because emails are easy to 'delete,' when speaking on the phone with someone isn't so easy to forget."

Cori says she doesn't feel burdened with Michelle's excessive needs. "Only when it's late at night and I'm tired and she is tired and we have to put her into bed and things aren't working well, or we are miscommunicating. Some tears are shed, then we joke and we get over it."

When it comes to Michelle's ability to cope with things, Cori praises her sister: "She is unbelievable. I have always said there were 2 ways she could have gone with the news of her incident and prognosis: into a great depression where she does nothing about it and mopes and cries, or keeping positive and living life to the fullest as best as she can. She took the high road - keeping positive – but sometimes I just don't know how she does it. Other than in the hospital as a precaution (and it didn't last long at all), she has never been on anti-depressants. She is a true inspiration! Whenever I get down and out, I think of her and 'suck it up'!"

When asked if she had ever put herself in Michelle's position, Cori says, "Yep, many times. I couldn't have done it. Her patience is amazing – when people talk loud because they think she is deaf, or people talk about her like she isn't even in the room, or she would like something done and has to wait from 10 to 45 minutes for it to get done, she keeps relatively calm. She is more than patient with everyone and everything. Me, I couldn't do it. I'd be angry and frustrated and have blow-ups all the time. Her situation is such a test and I'm not sure I would pass."

The tragic ordeal with Michelle has definitely changed Cori's way of looking at life. "Before Michelle's incident, I had never come across disability, no one with disabilities and if I had, I didn't know how to act around them. Since all of this, I am no longer afraid to talk to anyone. I make it a point to talk to everyone – all persons are human and deserve being treated like human beings. There are many lonely people in this world, and everyone deserves to have a friend. All of this has opened my eyes to a whole other world out there."

Cori's final comments relate to what she misses from Michelle before the stroke. "Really, the ability to spend time in the lake swimming and horsing around. I miss her being able to physically do things for herself, like get on a plane and come visit me at my house. I miss her voice – to hear it on the phone when we are so far away.

"I am so proud of her and her 'fight', of her accomplishments, of her painting, of her hope, of her constant determination to have a life. She is a hero, an angel."

Chapter 30

Michelle has answered a lot of questions over the past two years via email. I have made an effort to organize her thoughts into a commentary of her past, present and future.

Initially Michelle was very hesitant to speak of her personal life:

"I'm reading this and I don't know if I can do this. I have left out many details. When I had the stroke I lost, all, absolutely ALL privacy, and now I have to do that with my past?"

When asked to describe a day in her life when she lived at Creekside Landing she wrote:

"How incredibly boring, but OK. Around eight I turn TV on and eventually ring my call bell. The care aid eventually comes and turns off my bell and calls the nurse to hang about a litre of water mixed with half an ensure drink. I either have bowel care or I get a minimal wash and am dressed. Oh, Tuesday and Thursday morning from 9:30 to 10 I have the physiotherapist come do some general stretching while I'm still in bed. This is my biggest complaint. I no longer get any physio. I'm usually in my chair by 10:30 but then my shirt is changed, tray put on and computer set up. And it's most important that I'm positioned right in my chair. From eleven to noon I open email. At noon I go to the kitchen area for lunch. I'm usually the last one eating because I have to wait when other people need something. From one to five I watch TV and email or play Freecell on the computer, or do something on the computer. Five is dinner. From about six to eight I watch a movie and email. Cori usually texts me. About eight thirty I get another litre of water. When that is finished I go to bed. The care aid brushes my teeth and changes shirt for my pj tshirt. I have a button switch that controls my TV, a radio and a little lamp. So I watch TV

until eleven and then sleep with the radio on to drown out other noises. The next day I start over."

Michelle explains a bit about bowel care and general body cleansing, something a lot of people are curious about:

"Every Monday, Wednesday and Friday I have bowel care. Like many spinal cord injuries my bowel doesn't work properly so I get a suppository three times a week and sit on my commode. The privates are washed daily but I only get one shower a week. Another reason I have a perm, I hate greasy hair. They lay me on the bed to dress me, then into my chair."

When asked about why it was chosen for her to have a permanent catheter rather than using diapers, Michelle explains:

"The catheter was more a medical issue to make sure I didn't get another bladder stone, and to protect my skin from sitting in a wet brief."

Speech therapy has been somewhat of a sore spot for Michelle over the years. Here are some of her comments:

"Yes, when I was at the Gorge Road Hospital I had speech therapy which included mouth exercises. The therapist retired and I was dropped. Dad often tells people that I slipped through the cracks and it's so true.

"I can't even pucker my lips intentionally. The exercises are basic tongue movement. Stick my tongue out, moving my tongue from side to side, and running my tongue over my teeth and up to roof of my mouth. Sounds so minor but I can't always do it.

"For me it's easier to say anything in bed. Yes vocal cord is fine. It's getting enough airflow. Maybe it's the lack of muscle control? No, I don't have any speech therapy. The only explanation for no help is that it's all money based. Like eighty bucks and hour.

"Speech is something that will always bother me. I'm sure if speech therapy had continued I could speak by now.

"It's funny because now apparently I'm far more vocal and sometimes even understood. Yes, I hate the sound but I think I will just have to get over it."

Michelle describes her problems with eyesight:

"There are a few things I never bother to mention. They can't be helped or fixed so I just endure it. Like my vision. I had some physio but I don't have

great vision and maybe never will. I have slight double vision and bad perception. I hate sidewalks because my depth perception is so off I'm afraid of rolling off the edge."

There have been various problems Michelle has had to deal with over the years. She discussed some of them in her emails:

"One of the first things I noticed is how people talk over you. I still get that.

"There were many days that part of my physio was just to sit up in my chair. I only handled about ten minutes initially and I really wondered what kind of stupid life was I in for. Tammi would come in with a new boyfriend and I really wished I wasn't stuck there.

"That happens (requiring assistance) even today when I can't reach the bell. Depends what I'm calling for. If it's something minor I might just go to sleep if at night. Usually I would cry. Eventually I would alert someone. It was humiliating to know you just can't help yourself.

"Another issue is staffing. I get absolutely stressed out with new or casual staff. In the hospital or a facility it happens often where regular staff call in sick. I have my whole routine written out for these occasions. Because I can't speak after the computer is off I really need it written out. I get so tired of explaining and writing everything for young, impatient care aids. I really try to be patient, they don't know better.

"The biggest issue I have is in knowing all I lost and to know what I am missing out on every day. I used to be adventurous and outgoing but now I'm more cautious and have trust issues. The best example of this is that I almost had my pilot license and now I'm very afraid of heights.

"I went to Kamloops for Christmas. It's always a split occasion when I'm home because I love it and I know that Mom and Dad do everything for me but I feel like I'm three again."

Michelle often mentions issues she has experienced when joining her family on outings:

"The last two years we all go up to Sunpeaks for four days. It's good family time at the ski hill and I get to go skiing. It really does sound great. It's good for almost everyone. I feel selfish to even think it but I often have an

overwhelming sense of being left out. I can't get into any room so I sleep on the hide-a-bed in the living room and my brother just lifts me onto the bed. I never have any privacy.

"I can't use the hot tub or steam shower so I drink alcohol not to feel the cold so much. During this time alcohol is my friend."

Michelle described her adventures, long before her stroke, in Banff:

Ahhh Banff. Fun summer. Tammi and I were the first females to work in the dish room. This included cleaning out the huge vats permanently fixed in the kitchen and other cleaning or sorting jobs. This was technically a work term for school but a very social time. After a week it felt like home and there was always something to do. The dish room was a pretty brainless job but we were able to see how each department interacted. We also worked as banquet servers. There was somehow time to play. Many nights Tammi and I went to the pub or bar with some of the others. There were two or three main bars but we often started at one of the many pubs or restaurants. We lived in staff accommodation at the Rimrock hotel up Sulphur Mountain near the base of the gondola. There was a staff cafeteria but finding a decent meal was few and far between. There was usually fresh soup daily but different meals were plated and in a like vending machine. Each employee had a card with so many points daily for food. It also had a pop machine. I met many people and many guys. The first thing I noticed was cute guys everywhere. I had driven out there from Vernon with my other friend, Tanya, but we didn't hang out much. She worked in the restaurant as a server and met other people. Tammi and I became good friends and soon met Donny and Mark. They were pilots in the Air Force going from Comox to Saskatoon.

"Tammi's very sincere and fun and practical. She has always been there for me since Banff. She used to do my nails for years and highlight my hair."

In one email Michelle told me a bit about her personality as a teenager:

"My younger me: I was always very nice. I can't imagine not always being polite and courteous. I always smiled and often laughed. I think self-centered because I don't remember so much. Many little things. There was one girl in our

high school class in a wheelchair. I always thought I was nice enough but I didn't have a clue. Now I understand why she always looked a little angry. I don't even know what caused the wheelchair."

Michelle explains a bit about her personal emotions:

"I had a blink board so I could spell out words. My family and friends knew me and did lots of filling in the blanks. Cori was especially good and Dad didn't have much patience for it. I quickly learned that expressions said lots and tears definitely said lots. Communication really isn't vocal but lot of emotion and how I felt never got discussed. I think not upsetting me was a big part of not discussing emotion but I have never been a big talker when it's personal. Obviously. Hehe. Even now Cori and I cry together."

"I was thinking about more emotion. I don't think can do it. Sure, there are times I just ache not to be in a chair. I hate not being able to do dishes or bake or drive or simply to talk, but I can't dwell on that or I'd go insane. I have my painting and everything I CAN do.

Michelle talks about dealing with her limitations and trying to improve the quality of her life:

"Now I feel everything, normal on the right and harder to distinguish on the left side. Any little improvements were great.

"Now I can move my neck, so I raise eyes for yes and shake my head for no. It's far less blinking and more recognized to the public. The computer is Morse code. It's best because even outside I can type without really being able to see the screen. Morse code is second nature now.

"My taste is very normal. Which made not eating even worse.

"After about eight months my Dad really went to bat for me and fought to allow me to eat orally. I had slowly been reducing feeds put into the hanging bag because I was so full and afraid of gaining weight, however, I had to laugh at the first lunch meal I ever had. Mom and Dad fed me the couple of teaspoons of food brought in the tiny ketchup dispensing cups."

Michelle was asked how she managed to cope with things and what she thought of her future:

"Even after the stroke I was alive and really believed I could do anything. I still believe there is more for me. Maybe that is why I'm game to try most

things. I often wonder what I would be doing if I didn't have a stroke. But if I didn't have the stroke I never would have met so many wonderful people.

"I secretly think my life was going down a weird path and this was a definite way to change that. I even used to think if I truly changed I would get better. Now…I really don't know but I really miss the person I was.

"I hate when people go on and on about an injury or illness. I don't want it to define me.

"Eventually I grew a thick skin to all the stares I got. It bothered me for a long time. I didn't mind kids being curious and some even asked me about my computer or what happened. I can't believe how many adults rudely stare. I could never figure out why they just didn't ask.

"I seriously don't know how I cope. I cry a hell of a lot, almost daily. Almost every evening I put a movie on and close the door to escape. Oh, and light off. Even after ten years I don't feel like this will be the rest of my life. There are too many robotics, technical and medical advances going on. I think in about five years there could be a breakthrough."

Michelle explains her feelings about the time she had been living at Creekside Landing and dealing with an institutionalized environment:

"I think that is why so far Vernon (Creekside) *bothers me so much. I'm not living. I'm existing. And that isn't right. I often think it was great that I did so much. Being Gemini I have two ways of looking at this. I can do almost anything. I just need to be creative sometimes. Like in Victoria I had strong male caregivers so sometimes if the situation arose they could just carry me. The other 'me' is maybe in denial, maybe a strong belief that there will be some medical breakthrough in the next five, ten years. I don't plan to be so disabled for the rest of my life.*

"I liked Victoria (condo) *and Kelowna* (apartment) *because I was able to be me. I had the freedom to be me. I wasn't Gordon's daughter or Paul's sister. Vernon is really nice to have family close but I have no individuality. I rely on them too much.*

"Well obviously physically stuck and stuck at Creekside but more than that. I had a roommate (before the stroke) *in Victoria with MS. She was*

in a wheelchair but could walk a little. Her days were spent in her room and I'd often go out. Now I'm that person. I never used to be afraid of heights; now even watching someone on a building roof on TV makes my toes curl. Actually going back is good because I can see how far I've come. I get anxious in that my world is getting too closed in.

"Well, I'm presently stuck. I really liked Kelowna better but my brother and his family live here. I have a cute two year old niece and new month old nephew.

"Ya, Mom and Dad have had enough. They tried to discourage me (from moving) *but I have no other choice unless I did have a million kicking around. Cori and Paul are really busy so here I sit.*

"I think I'm going to find a counsellor. My brother and I were talking last night. After ten years I'm still not at peace with this and feel stuck.

"This has probably been the hardest year of my life but something has to improve eventually. I don't even think of suicide much. To me that is such a cop out. If I learned anything from Scott it was how to make the most of what you have. I think of all the people I do know that love me. Suicide would just hurt not help."

When asked how she would have dealt with Cori having the stroke instead of herself, Michelle wrote:

"Now there is a thought. I would be horrified of course but I don't know that I would be so constantly supportive. It's been almost twelve years she has helped keep me sane. I don't know if I would have done that."

Michelle reflects on the passing of time:

"Time is something that amazes me constantly. In the hospital everything is pretty much routine. The days are very similar. I remember Dad used to read to me to help pass time. I didn't eat orally so I really just lied in bed hour after hour.

"It's amazing what really matters before the real world hits. Even now I seem to work at a slower pace."

When discussing religion and faith, Michelle says:

"Well, currently I'm really not religious. I always keep an open mind and I'm influenced by friends. In Kelowna I was friends with the pastor at

Mountainview. He was Lutheran. I often went to any of his seminars. In Victoria I found a church I liked. It was Presbyterian. I really liked the social aspect of church and school. I still go at Christmas and sometimes Easter either with Mom and Dad at United church in Kamloops or here with Paul and Jenn at United church. I'm more spiritual than religious.

"Religion has always been in my life but now my fundamental belief is shattered. How could this happen and why?

"I don't have much relationship with God. "

When it comes to education, Michelle comments very briefly:

"I learned more seemingly practical things by travel and working. Anyone can memorize a book. I was always a good student but never really saw the point, which is interesting now since I'm not really using it."

I asked Michelle if she ever had any dreams:

"I rarely dream, but I'm always walking and talking when I do."

Physical activities for Michelle are something she aspires to and organizes as often as she can with the help of family and friends:

"Victoria, capital health Region, had a bigger health budget I think. I lived in a townhouse with CSIL funding so I had my own caregiver 24-7 and a roommate I barely saw. I was rarely home and actually had friends. There is really so much I can do with help and work. I have been hiking, kayaking, sailing, camping. Sometimes you have to be creative and it definitely helped having a fit, male caregiver.

"Skiing is fun. I dress in front of everybody immediately into my snow pants. I don't ski until one but I'm going into my chair so have to be dressed appropriately. When it's time, Dad and Cori drive me a couple of minutes to the day lodge where I used to work. We meet Gord, and Cori helps me get my gear on; gear being my winter jacket, toque, gloves and later my neck brace and scarf. I don't bring my computer with me. Apparently I have very expressional eyes. I get pushed to the outside and lifted from my chair to a sit ski."

Michelle was asked some philosophical questions:

My purpose? I'm not sure. I have my painting and hope soon to have my website going. I'm waiting for my brother's help to register my domain name.

I need so much help with everything, I don't know. That is also why I think hyperbaric oxygen therapy could help even improve my painting.

I don't have any regrets. You name it, I've done it. Except have children.

'What is the meaning of life? Who knows? I have considered this with and without religion. Either way, I have no answers. Why did this happen to me? What made me the lucky one?

Finally, I asked Michelle to write the closing paragraph of this book… her book:

Even now it amazes me how important communication is. I'm conscious of not answering questions, even with the use of a computer. There are usually three reasons for this; it depends who's asking, I'm already typing something, or I'm not sure how to answer. Sometimes I find the person really doesn't care what the answer is and has continued on with conversation. The computer can't portray sarcasm or any other inflection. My face apparently is very expressive and I don't even have to say things sometimes. That is beneficial, but maybe I should be more stoic sometimes.

I've had a few conversations today that have me thinking. I now live in my own townhouse and am finally done my fight. Sure, there will always be funding and supplies needed but I'm not in a hospital and I'm not in a facility. I'm reminded of my first trip to Australia. I'm free.

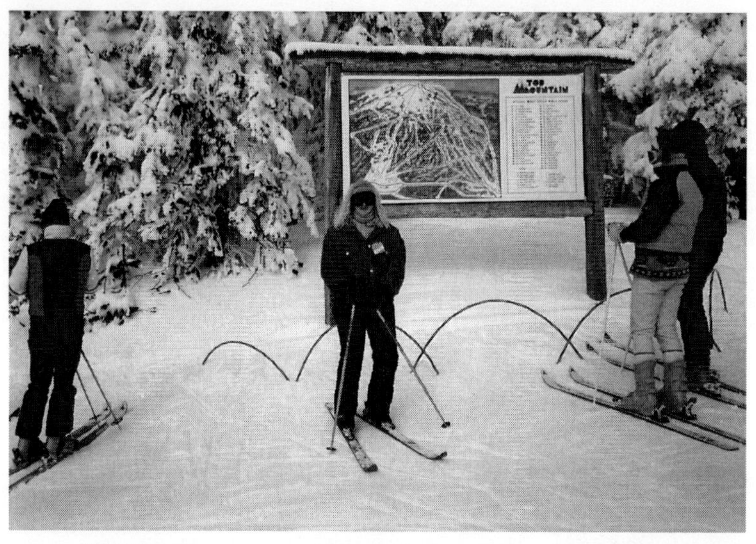

(1989 MICHELLE AT TODD MOUNTAIN BEFORE IT WAS CALLED SUNPEAKS)

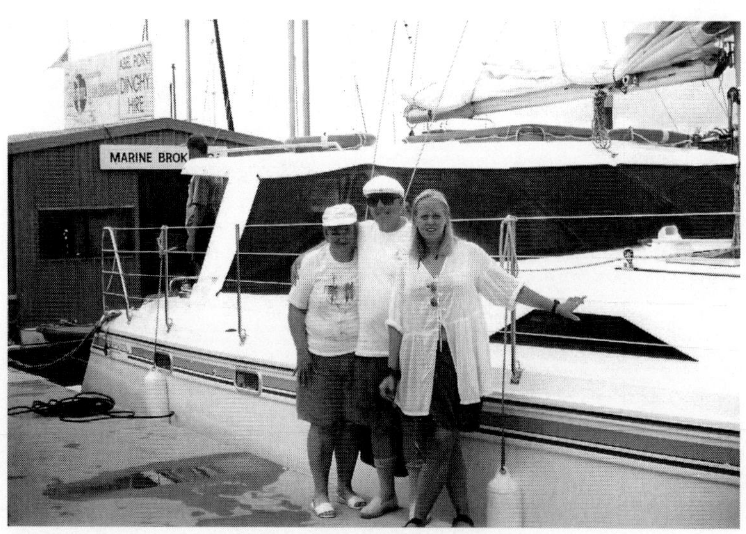

(1996 MICHELLE AND HER PARENTS, JOAN AND GORDON, IN AUSTRALIA)

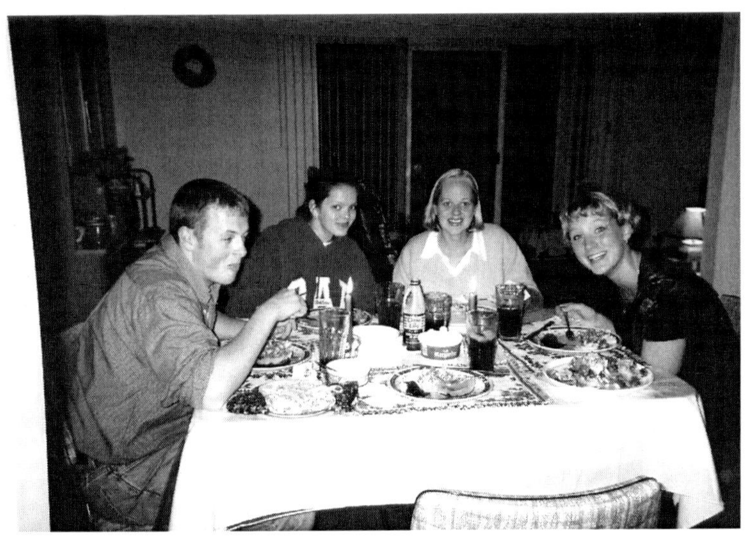

(1998 FROM LEFT TO RIGHT, PAUL, JENN, MICHELLE, AND TAMMI AT THE BEAR STREET TOWNHOUSE IN VICTORIA)

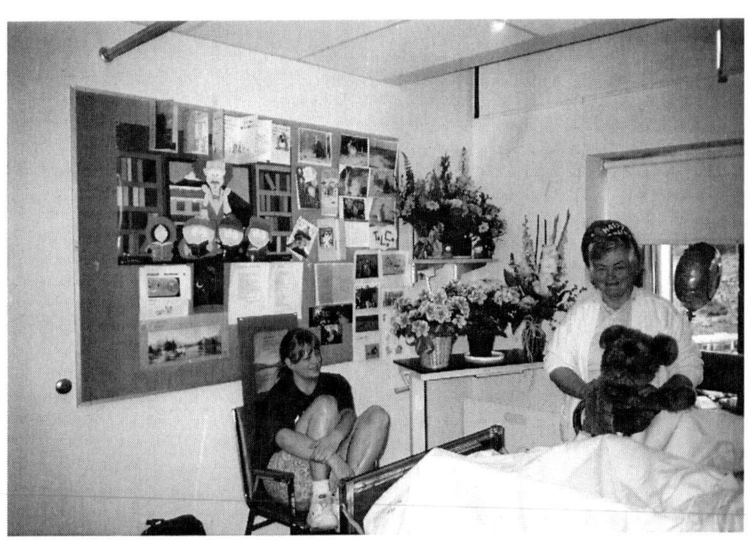

(1999 JOAN AND CORI AND MICHELLE IN THE FIRST HOSPITAL ROOM AT VICTORIA GENERAL HOSPITAL AFTER MICHELLE'S 25 BIRTHDAY)

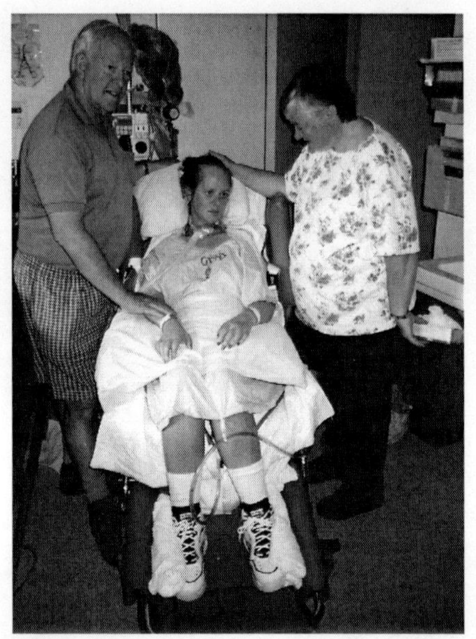

(2000 JOAN AND GORDON WITH MICHELLE, HER FIRST TIME IN HER CHAIR AT VICTORIA GENERAL HOSPITAL)

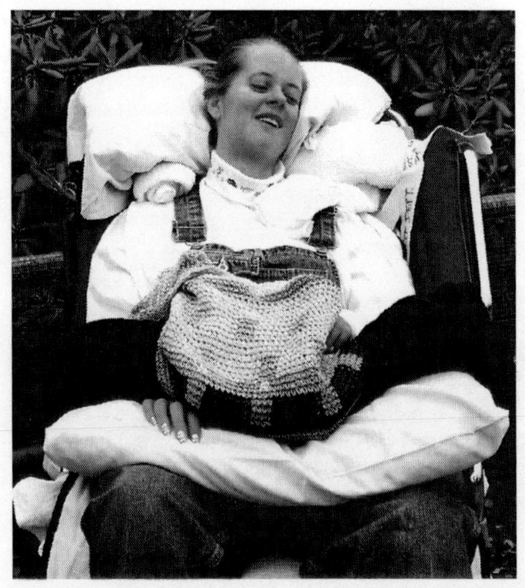

(2000 MICHELLE'S FIRST VENTURE OUTSIDE THE HOSPITAL)

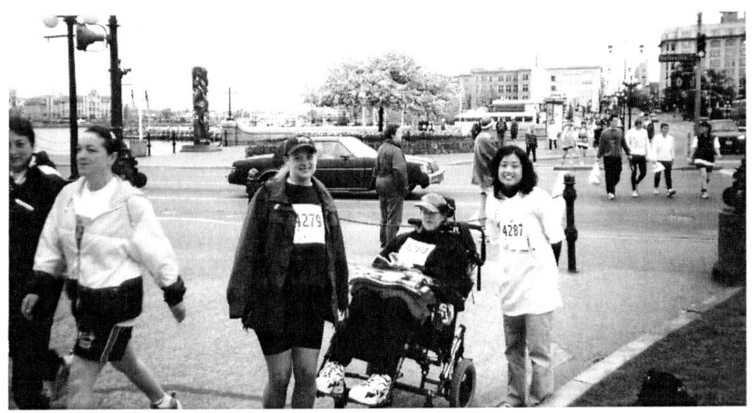

(2000 CORI, MICHELLE AND A FRIEND IN THE TIMES COLOMNIST 10K RUN IN VICTORIA)

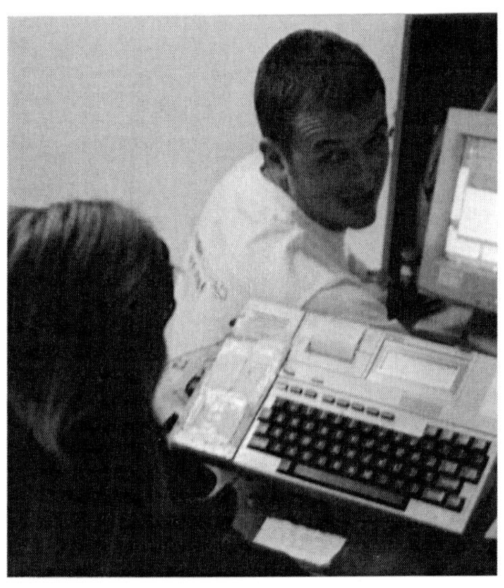

(2001 PAUL AND MICHELLE WITH THE EPSON COMPUTER)

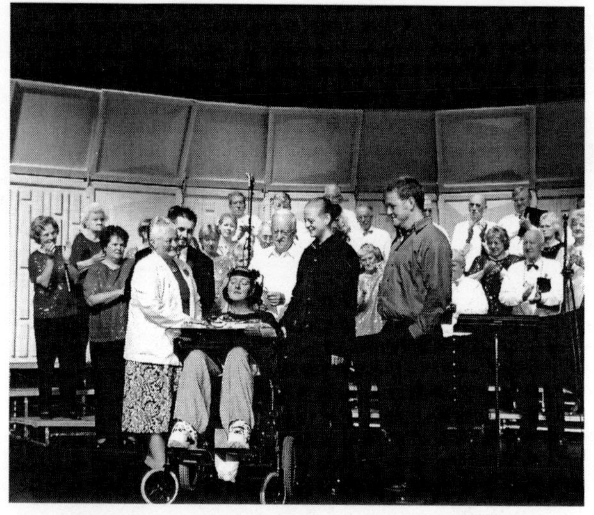

(2003 CHORAL FESTIVAL, MICHELLE'S FUNDRAISER IN KAMLOOPS. JOAN, CORI, AND PAUL WITH MICHELLE ONSTAGE)

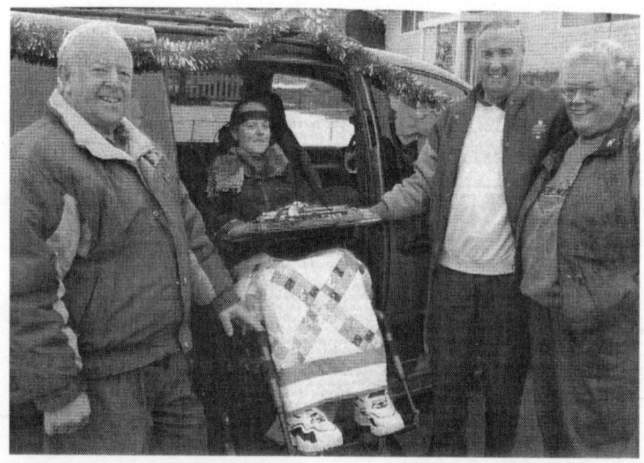

(2003 MICHELLE'S NEW VAN, PURCHASED AFTER THE FUNDRAISER IN KAMLOOPS. GORDON AND GOOD FAMILY FRIEND, MR. DOVE)

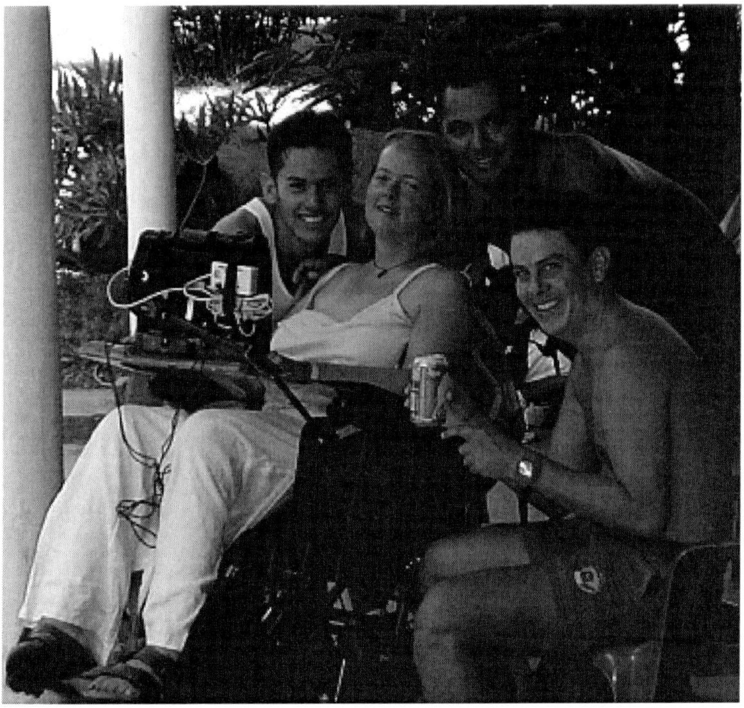

(2003 MICHELLE AND SOME MEXICAN MEN FROM THE HOTEL IN PUERTO VALLARTA. SHE SEEMS TO ATTRACT EVERYONE WITH HER CONTAGIOUS SMILE!)

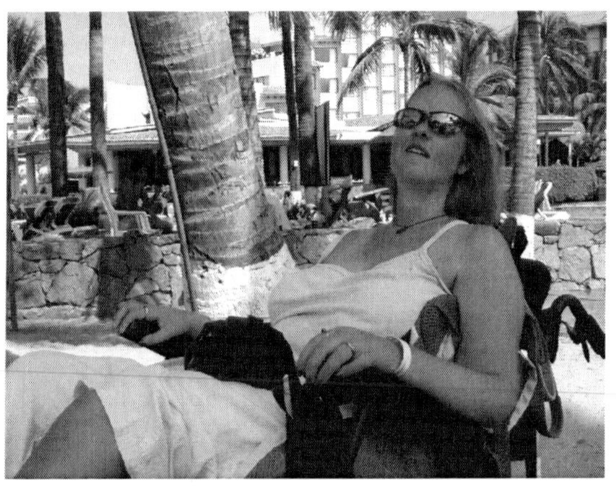

(2003 MICHELLE RELAXING IN MEXICO!)

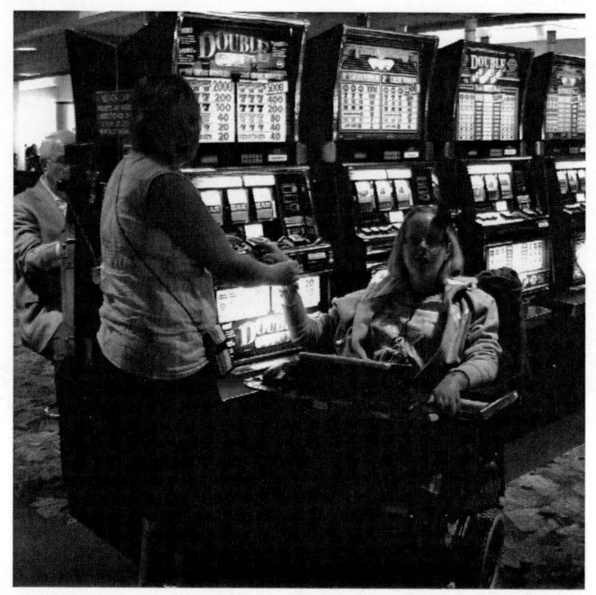

(2009 MICHELLE PLAYING THE SLOTS IN LAS VEGAS WITH HER SISTER, CORI)

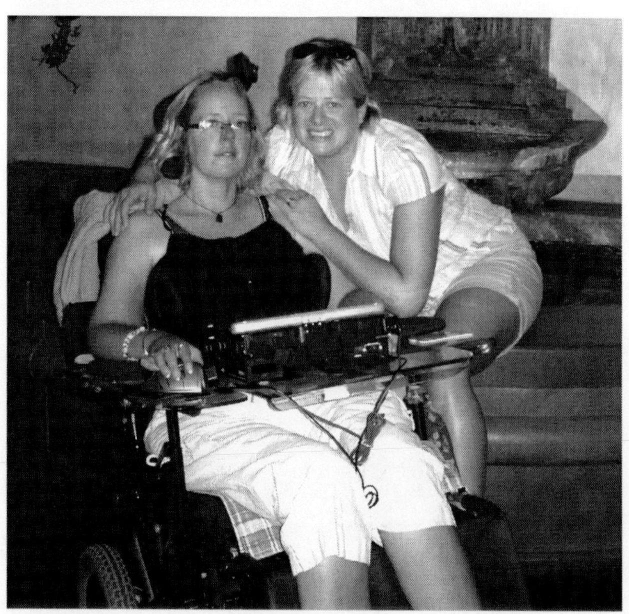

(2009 MICHELLE AND CORI IN THE PARIS HOTEL IN LAS VEGAS)

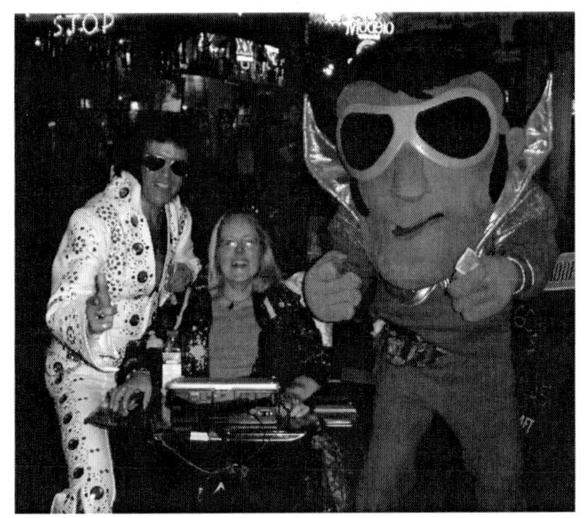

(2009 MICHELLE CELEBRATING WITH ELVIS IN LAS VEGAS!)

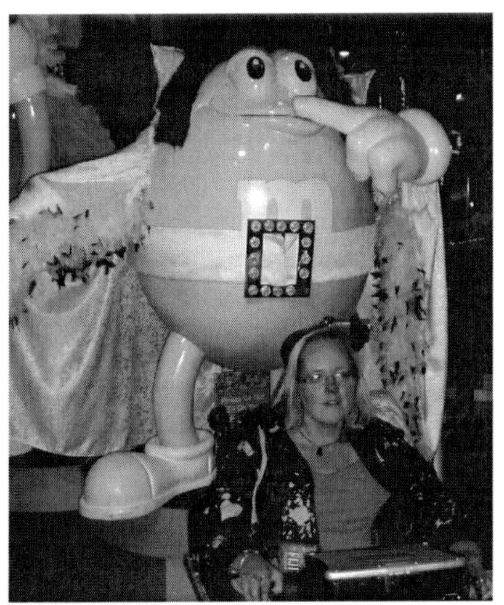

(2009 MICHELLE LIVING IT UP IN LAS VEGAS!)

Author's Note

It was on a "tag along" trip up to Vernon with BCPA consultant, Arlene Pilgrim, that I first met Michelle Britton. Arlene explained to me that we were going to visit a young woman who was paralyzed from the mouth down. According to Arlene, Michelle was an unusual case, one of the most disabled people Arlene had ever dealt with. And Arlene had vast experience with people in wheelchairs who had spinal cord injuries caused by an array of tragic events. Arlene expressed how unique Michelle was; how she maintained a good sense of humor despite her insurmountable disabilities.

Similar to most other folks, I was initially uncomfortable with Michelle. Her disability was profound. She was unable to speak. She raised her eyes upwards to greet us. To use Michelle's own words, she did look rather "freakish." Her wheelchair was heavy duty with fairly large, well-treaded wheels and a motor under the seat. She had all sorts of contraptions at her disposal, all within reach of her right hand. Her computer rested on a tray in front of her. Michelle had little expression on her face. Her head did not move and was supported in the back by a special headrest that not only held her head from behind but also had a brace on the side. Michelle was very, very disabled.

I stood on the sidelines and observed Arlene's interaction with Michelle. When Arlene asked a question, Michelle would look quickly upwards for an affirmative answer. For a negative reply she would slowly move her head from side to side, very slowly. If Michelle wanted to say anything she would begin to tap away with her index finger at a button situated on the right side of her tray. There was a half-ball shaped gadget that she rested her hand upon, probably to keep her hand in a comfortable position for her single finger movement. Within her reach was also a tiny lever with a little ball on the end. This was for controlling her motorized wheelchair. It was quite the setup.

It was clear to me that Michelle relied very heavily on computers and motorized equipment. But everything with Michelle was slow going. It would take several seconds for her to type one word. An entire sentence of about ten words would take her a couple of minutes. It dawned on me just how incredibly fast verbal communication is for the rest of us. Michelle's reality was that of operating at a snail's pace. Yet, rather than my feeling frustrated with her slowness, I found myself beginning to relax. That was a surprise.

When I went home from that memorable trip, I mentioned Michelle to a couple of friends. They would mostly have that same look on their face when I spoke of Michelle's circumstances, that blank stare, that thoughtful expression of horror. When I couldn't stop thinking about her I knew I had to write about her. This is a story that needed to be told.

With Michelle's permission and her parent's blessing, I embarked on my first biography. And I was so fortunate right from the very beginning. Michelle's family had kept daily diaries for nearly two years during Michelle's ordeal. The diaries led me into the depths of a young woman's journey that nobody should ever have to live through.

The two huge diaries containing hundreds of pages of comments and information from Michelle's hospital stay had been kept in storage for almost a decade. The first time I met Michelle's parents, Joan and Gordon, was at Creekside Landing, the care facility where Michelle lived when I met her. It really was a nice place, but it was so much like a hospital, spotlessly clean, and it smelled of disinfectant, like a hospital. And my sense when I entered the building was that of lingering ill-health, like this was a place of finality, a place to be warehoused until life ended.

On the other hand, the planners of Creekside Landing had done their best to make it a place with a few uplifting comforts. The main living room area was nicely furnished and well decorated including attractive pictures on the walls. There was a large fish tank with colorful varieties of fish actively fluttering through the water. A door on one wall led to a nicely stocked library with a few chairs and a round table. This is where I conducted my interview with Joan and Gordon. Michelle was present.

I felt quite at ease with the Brittons. It was occasionally difficult for them to go back in time and relive the agony of Michelle's first few weeks in the hospital. Joan often spoke through tears. Gordon remained stoic and matter of fact, yet, would once in a while go into a contemplative silence. There was such tremendous pain behind his quiet face.

The interview lasted about an hour and a half. Through this meeting I learned so much about the relationship between mother, dad and daughter. Joan displayed all the characteristics of a nurturing mom, touching Michelle's arm and shoulder, sweeping a loose strand of hair from her face. When Gordon spoke to his daughter he endearingly called her Shell.

The diaries were invaluable. Here was an every-day account of Michelle's desperate journey written in the hands of those who were right there. Michelle herself could not recall much of what happened to her, especially in those first few weeks. And, to make things even better, I discovered that Michelle herself had written a few diaries of her vacations when she was younger. I could not believe my good fortune. Now I had her thoughts and feelings as a young healthy person, the Michelle before the stroke.

Getting to know Michelle was not difficult. Communicating with her via email was easy and fun. Her replies were smart, humorous, and witty, but as always, frustratingly brief. One must always keep in mind that she types by using Morse code and, although this is much faster that using a blink board, it is still not the same as the flying fingers of a 100 word per minute keyboarder. Michelle chooses her words sparingly.

The relationship between Michelle and her family is so interesting to observe. I was invited to Michelle's 36th birthday celebration at her brother's place. The first thing I noticed was that Paul's house was completely set up for wheelchair access with a ramp leading into the front door. Gordon and Joan brought Michelle over in her van. Gordon pulled out the ramp and carefully guided Michelle in her wheelchair down to the sidewalk. It wasn't a scene where there was any noticeable stress. Everyone seemed to carry on with the event as if there was nothing unusual, that having a severely handicapped family member among them was…normal. But then, it was normal. This was their life.

Jenn, Paul's wife, and Joan watched over the two children. Paul was busy barbequing hamburgers. And Gordon was stirring a thickening powder into a glass of beer. I watched as he patiently moved the spoon through the bronze liquid, adding a small amount of powder, then stirring; then adding more powder until the texture was just right. He then took the glass over to Michelle and began to hand feed her; a father calmly spoon-feeding his 36-year-old daughter a beer. I watched, fascinated.

When the hamburgers were ready, Joan put together a bun and burger along with all the condiments. She dumped the whole works into a blender. It was turned into an unappetizing glob. She scooped up a bit of hamburger mush into a spoon and fed it to Michelle. This was obviously their routine. Joan asked her something I didn't quite catch. Michelle looked upwards. Joan shook a few more drops of ketchup and mustard into the blender and mixed it up. She poured it into a bowl and set it on the table in front of Michelle where Gordon proceeded to feed her. He would take a bite of his own burger, and then he would give a spoonful of goop to Michelle.

To me it all seemed a bit out of the ordinary. To them it was simply another average family gathering.

The kids accepted Michelle as if there were absolutely nothing unusual about their wheelchair-bound aunt. The baby, of course, was too young to pay much mind, but little Emery, now over two years old, was quite aware of Michelle and was very used to the wheelchair and her very quiet auntie.

The entire family sat around the table eating hamburgers and salad. It was a comfortable moment. There were lots of chatter and laughter. I noticed that Michelle was quietly observing, enjoying. I could tell there was clearly a good degree of quality to her life.

Over the months that I slowly got to know the family, I found that witnessing Michelle with Cori was emotionally uplifting. To see the complete bonding love between sisters makes you feel…good. Cori runs around her sister's new home, efficiently placing notes here and there so that care givers know about important things in Michelle's daily needs. It is the end of a long visit. Cori has spent most of the summer with her sister, but she must now return to Calgary, to her family. It has been a struggle for Cori. She needs to be close to Michelle. She has decided to move back to Vernon. It is a complicated choice. Her husband will join her. His children: maybe. It is a struggle.

If I have learned anything from writing this book it is that the quality of a person's life depends on access to some sort of funding, especially if that person is totally disabled and in need of expensive care.

Because of the lack of funding, Michelle has spent a good portion of her post-stroke life living/existing in institutions. Her personal care has been outstanding. In Canada, our care of persons with disabilities is stellar when compared with most other countries in the world. However, we, the able bodied people in our society, are comfortable with merely providing the best physical care possible, while we definitely fall short in giving a disabled person a certain degree of independence, and control over their daily living.

I now realize how terribly lost Michelle would be without technical assistance. Given the extremely limited condition in which Michelle now exists, I can't help but wonder what her life would have been like had her situation happened twenty or thirty years ago. Despite not being able to move her limbs; stand, walk, speak, Michelle enjoys unlimited access to the world around her. With her computer she is able to connect regularly with friends and family. Before the internet became a common tool, this would have been impossible. With the technical and medical advances of each decade, Michelle can take advantage of improving her life in small but helpful ways.

I am happy for Michelle. She is very content living in her own home, taking charge of her life. To have an uncooperative body along with a high functioning mind is her daily challenge. I know from communicating with Michelle that she wants to enjoy every minute of her life. She wants to experience adventure, take in the wonders of the world around her; absorb the love of her family and her friends. Michelle wants to live.